LUPUS Q&A

LUPUS Q&A

. . . .

Everything You Need to Know

. . . .

REVISED EDITION

Robert G. Lahita, M.D., Ph.D.

and

Robert H. Phillips, Ph.D.

AVERY

a member of
Penguin Group (USA) Inc.
375 Hudson Street
New York, New York 10014
www.penguin.com

Copyright © 1998, 2004 by Robert G. Lahita and Robert Phillips
Previously published as *Lupus: Everything You Need to Know*

LIBRARY OF CONGRESS CATALOGING-IN-PUBLICATION DATA

Lahita, Robert G. (Robert George), date.
Lupus Q&A : everything you need to know / Robert G. Lahita
and Robert H. Phillips.—Rev. ed.
p.   cm.
Rev. ed. of: Lupus
Includes index.
ISBN 1-58333-196-4
1. Systemic lupus erythematosus—Popular works.   I. Phillips, Robert H., 1948–
II. Lahita, Robert G. (Robert George), 1945– Lupus.   III. Title.
RC924.5.L85L34   2004   2004040974
616.7'72—dc22

Printed in the United States of America
1   3   5   7   9   10   8   6   4   2

Book design by Amanda Dewey

Contents

Foreword

It is my great pleasure to write a foreword to this book, dedicated to the patient with lupus and written by Dr. Robert Lahita, who has done so much for my family, in conjunction with Dr. Robert Phillips.

Autoimmune disease, a topic that is very important to my family, can strike anyone at any age. One of the great mysteries of our time, this category of illness inflicts psychological and physical damage upon its sufferers. Systemic lupus erythematosus, in particular, has caused untold devastation and suffering for lupus patients and their families. It is also a disease that is harder to diagnose than it is to pronounce. This is why it is important to have a book like this one—solid and comprehensive, yet simple and direct. It answers questions for patients, for their families, and perhaps even for their doctors. The authors have taken particular aim at the public interest in this disease that affects women most, but has an impact on people of every gender, of every age, and of every race; and in doing so have given some attention and interest to a disease that affects many but about which so little is known. I know, for this disease has touched, and will doubtless continue to touch, the members of my family.

George joins me in wishing all patients and their families well and in hoping that *Lupus Q & A: Everything You Need to Know* will help many people to understand and cope with this dreaded disease.

BARBARA BUSH
Former First Lady
Houston, Texas

Preface

There is no more difficult disease to diagnose, understand, or treat than the disease called *systemic lupus erythematosus*. This may be due to the fact that lupus is not one disease but many diseases grouped under one heading. It may also be because the disease can present itself to both physicians and patients in mysterious ways; throwing them off the track, leading them to think of other more common illnesses, and eluding standard diagnostic methods. Whatever the reason, lupus is complex and problematic.

This book was designed to answer the many questions you may have about this disease and its impact on your life. Many of the questions are based on the countless numbers of patients who enter our clinics and offices daily with long lists of questions, the letters that arrive weekly in the mail seeking answers, the questions we hear at conventions or meetings, or the sad phone messages that ask for help because "my doctors don't understand the disease." This is not a companion to any textbook. It is written strictly for patients and is based on their needs and questions. The goal was not to educate doctors with the material in this book (although many will find it helpful) but rather to address patients' very real questions. We also realize that despite the dozens of questions answered in the book, the likelihood remains that certain areas may have been inadvertently overlooked. However, our goal was to address those questions that, according to our experience, are most on the minds of our patients.

Ironically, the disease lupus seems to have gotten more complex, not less, over the years. New knowledge about the immune system and its workings has led to other autoimmune diseases being added to the roster of problems that need resolution. For example, because of difficulties in classification, a disease such as autoimmune phospholipid syndrome is often given the label "lupus." Some physicians label it lupus in order to give the disease a billing code acceptable for insurance reimbursement! Diseases such as autoimmune phospholipid syndrome have resulted in swelling numbers of lupus patients. The Lupus Foundation of America has estimated that some 2 to 2.5 million Americans believe that they have lupus, and that some 86 percent of Americans have heard of the disease. While these are staggering numbers, one must be cautioned to remember that they may, at least to some degree, reflect the fact that many illnesses that are not lupus are being called lupus. Hopefully, this book will help to clarify the reasons that the numbers of people with lupus are increasing.

Last, a bit of history is necessary to allow readers to understand this disease and its past. Let's review the "time-line" of lupus.

- Lupus got its name because it was originally thought to represent the wounds that would result from being attacked by a wolf. The trademark "butterfly rash" was thought to be from the bite or scratches of a wolf.
- This butterfly rash on the malar part of the face (above the cheeks) was first mentioned in the thirteenth century.
- The actual term *lupus erythematosus* was first mentioned by a fellow named Cazenavé in 1851.
- There was much confusion regarding the diagnosis of lupus until well into this century. It was often confused with tuberculosis, disseminated gonorrhea, and many skin disorders.
- Only in the 1930s and 1940s did pathologists look at organs like the kidneys and skin and realize that there were common changes in these organs that had certain similarities in patients with lupus. Together these formed the typical aspects of lupus.
- Immunology was in its infancy in the 1930s and 1940s, and the classical description of antibody structure was not to take place for

some decades. No one knew the mechanism through which lupus could so globally damage so many organs of the body. No one really understood this newly described illness, which counted rash, kidney failure, and sun sensitivity among its list of characteristics.

- In the 1940s came the association with the false positive test for syphilis, the discovery of the LE cell, and the idea that these phenomena might have something to do with "blood proteins." These proteins were later called antibodies, and it was suggested that they might be reacting with normal tissues. All of these discoveries were important in the understanding and diagnosis of lupus.

- Coincidentally, the discovery of cortisone in 1948 by Philip Hench provided the first and greatest therapy for lupus.

- The 1950s brought the fluorescent antinuclear antibody assay, an important test in the diagnosis of lupus, and the discovery of autoantibodies like Sm, RNP, and others. These autoantibodies form the basis for our understanding of the disease process of lupus—how we diagnose it and a small bit about how the disease affects the body. In addition, the 1950s brought about important insight into the genetics of the disease. All of this added significantly to the knowledge about lupus.

- Since the 1950s, much research has focused on the following areas: molecular genetics (in order to learn more about the immune response), hormones and their importance, and, more recently, the development of several new drugs. Although lupus research has come far in the past twenty-five years, it will take an understanding of the cause of the disease—currently unknown—in order to develop a targeted cure.

- In the early 1980s a new condition called antiphospholipid syndrome was described that in many cases is inexorably linked to lupus. It is very troubling because it causes bleeding and clotting. It is usually a condition of "sticky blood" that can result in blood clots in the lungs or the brain. The addition of factors concerning the syndrome resulted in a revision of the criteria for the classification of lupus.

Despite all of the early history of this disease, we have a long way to go in our understanding of lupus and related illnesses. However, we have made strides in the last twenty years that have revolutionized the way we examine many illnesses. Great discoveries are yet to happen. Let us hope that this book will continue to enlighten patients as we move ahead.

ROBERT LAHITA, M.D., PH.D.
LibertyHealth—Jersey City Medical Center
Jersey City, New Jersey

ROBERT H. PHILLIPS, PH.D.
Center for Coping
Long Island, New York

LUPUS Q&A

1.

LUPUS: AN OVERVIEW

. . . .

Lupus is a very complex disease that even the experts do not understand completely. So, of course, once patients are diagnosed with lupus, they have many questions about this puzzling disorder. This chapter will introduce you to the basics of lupus. First, we will answer the question "Just what is lupus?" We will then discuss the different types of lupus, the causes of the disease, and common myths surrounding the disorder.

THE NATURE OF LUPUS

What is lupus?

Lupus is an *autoimmune disease*. The immune system, which normally protects the body, turns against itself (*auto*) and attacks it. Lupus has no known cause and, as a result, no known cure. The disease can affect many different systems of the body, and there are many different ways that it can affect people.

Why is it called lupus?

In the early twentieth century, most physicians thought lupus was a skin disease. The disease got its name because many patients looked as though they had been bitten or scratched by wolves. *Lupus,* in Latin, means "wolf."

Why is lupus referred to as a chronic disease?

Lupus is considered a chronic disease because it is currently incurable. Once one experiences lupus symptoms, one has lupus forever. However, it should be noted that certain forms of lupus—such as the drug-related form—don't fit into this incurable category because once the drugs that have "caused" the lupus are withdrawn, the lupus symptoms go away.

Can lupus be both acute and chronic?

Yes. Lupus is a chronic disease but can have acute episodes. As a chronic disease, lupus often has a slow onset, and is ongoing and incurable. The immune system—unable to rid itself of what is perceived as a foreign substance—continues to react against the "foreign tissue." This can be a significant problem, lasting for quite a while—possibly up to many months—and can be accompanied by signs and symptoms of other chronic illnesses.

But a patient can experience acute episodes, times when symptoms can worsen in immediate, abrupt, and occasionally severe ways. These acute manifestations, known as "flares," can often occur this way, even in those who have had the disease for many years.

It's like a simmering pot of soup that all of a sudden bubbles over, or like a volcano that simmers and all of a sudden pops its lid, but then goes back down and simmers for another twenty years.

What is a connective tissue disorder?

This is the former name for lupus and other related diseases. In the past, any disorder involving the muscles, tendons, and, in some cases, even bones, used to be referred to as a connective tissue disease. It was once believed that the inflammation of connective tissue occurred only from overuse. We now know that connective tissue can be inflamed for a variety of reasons, some of which have nothing to do with overuse.

What is mixed connective tissue disease?

Mixed connective tissue disease is referred to as an "overlap syndrome" because there seems to be an overlap of several different diseases or symptoms, suggesting more than one disease. There are no specific signs or symptoms of overlap disease. To help doctors make this diagnosis, mixed connective tissue disease was originally associated with the presence of an antibody or specific protein in the blood called ribonucleoprotein antibody (RNP).

Some experts currently think that this overlap syndrome may be related more to a disease called scleroderma than to lupus. Many patients with lupus have the anti-RNP antibody, but one must have very high *titers,* or strength, of the antibody for mixed connective disease to be present. So the best way to describe mixed connective tissue disease is to call it a hybrid illness.

WHAT HAPPENS IN LUPUS

What exactly happens in lupus?

It is difficult to provide an accurate answer to this question. The key to understanding what happens in lupus is understanding the job of the immune system. The immune system is designed to protect the body from foreign invaders called *antigens.* The problem is that in lupus, the immune system cannot distinguish certain "self" tissues from foreign invaders and thus attacks inappropriate targets. So, for some reason, the immune system has a problem correctly identifying antigens and turns against the body that it is designed to protect.

What are the main components of the immune system?

The immune system is primarily made up of three categories of cells—the *B lymphocytes* (commonly called the *B cells*), the *T lymphocytes* (the *T cells*), and the *phagocytes*. These three groups of cells form the "soldiers" of the immune system, designed to protect the body from foreign invaders (antigens).

What exactly is an antigen?

Antigens are any substances, produced inside the body or coming from outside the body, that the immune system recognizes as being foreign—like germs, bacteria, viruses, or fungi. In other words, an antigen is any substance that can trigger an *immune response*—an effort made by the immune system to eliminate an unwanted foreign invader. In lupus, the immune system, suddenly, and for no apparent reason, turns against the body's own cells and tissues, mistaking them for foreign invaders, and tries to destroy them as it would other foreign matter. So the body is now reacting to *autoantigens* (self-antigens).

What is an autoantigen?

An *autoantigen* is a substance that occurs naturally within the body—in other words, it is not really foreign but is a "self" substance—but, for some reason, is identified by the immune system as foreign. The autoantigen then triggers an immune response, and the body fights it the way it would normally fight off foreign substances with *antibodies*. This is called an *autoimmune response*.

What are antibodies?

Antibodies are proteins that are among the five major classes of immunoglobulin molecules, protein molecules that work to kill foreign substances. They are produced by the immune system's B cells in response to the presence of the foreign substances (antigens), for the primary purpose of destroying them.

What are autoantibodies?

As you now know, antibodies are molecules that normally defend the body against foreign substances. *Autoantibodies* are the names for antibodies that fight healthy tissues within the body. The autoantibodies in no two patients have exactly the same target, although in families, two members with the disease may have autoantibodies that look very similar.

What do antibodies do?

Antibodies attach themselves to foreign substances until the combination of antibody and foreign substance (the *immune complex*) is engulfed by a scavenger cell, called a *phagocyte*. This cell usually digests the immune complex, destroying it. In some cases, after the immune complex is engulfed, the antibody and foreign agent go directly to the spleen to be deposited. The spleen is the depository or "graveyard" of old immune complexes. There are also cells in the spleen that are capable of engulfing and removing substances from circulation themselves.

What is an antigen–antibody reaction?

The *antigen-antibody reaction* is the process in the immune system that creates immune complexes. The white blood cells respond to an antigen by making antibodies. The antibody then binds with the antigen. An antigen is usually a foreign bacterium or virus in a healthy person. In a lupus patient, an antigen might be a clotting factor or a white cell.

What exactly is an immune complex?

Very simply, when the immune system reacts to an antigen, and antibodies attack it to destroy it, the attachment of antibody to antigen is called an *immune complex*.

What are lymphocytes?

Lymphocytes are the part of the white blood cell family that are produced in lymphoid tissue. They are the main cells of the immune system. There are different categories of lymphocytes, such as the killer cells and T and B cells. All of these cells have a purpose, such as attacking and swallowing, eliciting antibodies, or killing virus particles. These cells have amazing capabilities, and new functions of them are being discovered every year.

Since lupus is a disease of the immune system, lymphocytes play a major role—both in the manifestation of the disease and in the actual cause of illness. Their most important role in lupus is the production of antibodies.

What are T cells?

T cells stands for *thymus-derived lymphocytes*. There are several varieties of T cells. They can be "helper" cells (called the helper T cells) that help immune function by alerting the B cells to begin producing antibodies to fight off the antigens, "suppressor" cells that suppress immune function, or killer T cells (also called cytotoxic T cells) that recognize, attack, and destroy antigens.

Most of the T cells have certain markers on their surfaces, called *cluster determinants* or *CD* markers. They are usually given a number. There are about 170 CD markers. There are many researchers who have CD marker maps on their office walls because they are impossible to remember. These markers are important because they help us find subsets of lymphocytes. The subsets of lymphocytes are very important to know in a particular patient. Currently, they're used for diagnostic purposes. It is hoped that in the future they'll be used for therapeutic purposes.

CD markers were discovered for the first time with specific *monoclonal antibodies* (antibodies that are "tailor-made" in a laboratory in a mouse or in a cell culture). Monoclonal antibodies are not present in lupus patients. The monoclonal antibody is a way of learning more about these T cells in the laboratory. Essentially, the antibody was produced from an engineered fusion of two kinds of cells—a cancer cell and a normal immune cell. These antibodies are very highly specific and make great chemicals for study in the laboratory. Their "discoverers" were even awarded a Nobel prize.

What are B cells?

B cells (which received their name because they were discovered in the "bursa" part of the chicken gut) are very specialized lymphocytes that are responsible for a variety of functions. Their most important role, however, is their maturation into plasma cells and their eventual production of antibodies.

Do B cells come from the bursa in the human?

No, B cells do not come from a bursa in the human, but they are believed to come from the bone marrow, which is comparable to the bursa.

How does the immune system produce antibodies?

The immune system is programmed shortly after birth, or perhaps even before, to recognize certain antigens as "self" antigens. If a person is later exposed to an antigen that is not recognized as self, his or her immune system will reject it as foreign. This process of recognition goes on throughout life. When a person becomes infected with any organism, an immune response is made to that organism. After the initial reaction, there continues to be *immunological memory* for this foreign substance.

One goal of the immune system is the production of killer cells that are designed to counter any invasion of foreign viral materials. Another goal is the manufacture of antibodies. Antibodies engulf foreign substances and remove them from circulation.

In the immune system, there are T cells and B cells. The B cells are the cells that are responsible for making antibody. They can be stimulated to make antibody either by the foreign substance directly or by the T cells. When the B cells make antibody in response to stimulation by foreign matter, it is called a *T-independent response.* However, the T cells, also called the "helper or suppressor cells," can come along and stimulate the B cells themselves to make more antibody. These are called *T-dependent responses.*

What do T and B cells do?

The T cells recognize foreign invaders and respond by either killing them outright ("killer" T cells) or by presenting them to B cells so that a specific antibody can be made.

Describe the relationship between T lymphocytes and B lymphocytes.

This relationship is one of the most important ones of the immune system. The T cells remember previously identified antigens and usually activate themselves and the B cells. Antigens are usually recognized by what are called *antigen-presenting cells (APCs)* that are strategically placed in such parts of the body as the lungs, liver, and prostate. The APCs present the information, derived from a very complex process of recognition, to T cells. The T cell never forgets an antigen.

In a more complicated series of steps, antigens can also be directly presented to B cells. When a T cell is activated, it activates the B cells to respond to the antigen by specializing, or turning their efforts toward that foreign substance. This process is called *differentiation*. It allows the B cells to make antibodies that target the antigens. The amazing nature of this response has dazzled scientists for years and is still not fully understood.

What are phagocytes?

Phagocytes (also called accessory cells because they assist in the immune response) are white blood cells that can destroy certain particles or debris. The name *phagocyte* comes from the Greek *phagos,* to eat.

What are macrophages?

Macrophages are large, mature phagocytes. They have a number of important functions. They can, without any additional signal from the immune system, ingest and destroy foreign invaders, diseased cells, or cellular debris. They can also send signals to lymphocytes to alert them that antigens are present. They can also produce different *cytokines* (messengers to the immune system that facilitate the immune response).

What is complement?

Complements are special proteins in the blood that help the antibodies in their effort to rid the body of the antibody-antigen combination (the immune complex). They are so named because they complement, or enhance, the function of the immune system.

When an antigen is identified by the immune system as requiring destruction, and an antibody attaches to it, this triggers a chain reaction called a *complement cascade.* In this chain reaction, a series of complement components that are normally inactive in the blood become activated and come to the assistance of the antibody in eliminating the antigen.

A category of markers for lupus are called complement components. There are nine components of complement, which as a whole serve as amplifiers of the immune reaction. In other words, complement makes the immune reaction more efficient. Deficiencies in any of the nine complement components results in a derailment of efficient immune system functioning. (We discuss complement in more detail in chapter 2.) For some reason, when a person is deficient in some of the early components of complement, a lupus-like condition can be acquired. Such components include C2, C4, and C1Q.

What are leukocytes?

Leukocytes are white blood cells. When they receive the signal of invasion, they secrete chemicals, in an attempt to kill the antigens that cause the joint pain and swelling when a lupus patient goes into a flare. They can also be involved in the process of destroying foreign invaders. Leukocytes can be involved in causing many problems in lupus, such as pulmonary hypertension, rashes on the face, or the breakdown of lung tissue. They can also be stimulated by a variety of agents or complexes (like immune complexes).

Why is lupus an inflammatory disease?

Inflammation is a reaction of tissues to infection, injury, or invasion. It is usually characterized by swelling, redness, pain, heat, and reduced function. In lupus, inflammation is usually a result of an immune system reaction. The immune system believes one of the otherwise healthy tissues in the body is the foreign invader, and reacts accordingly, triggering the immune reaction that results in inflammation.

How does inflammation occur?

Inflammation is the result of a series of very well-engineered chemical reactions, involving many molecules called *mediators.* An immune reaction occurs when an antigen is recognized. The white blood cells, specifically the lymphocytes, generally trigger a signal that is sent to cells that contain the mediators. This signal triggers the release of the mediators.

The powerful mediators then cause all of the pain, the redness, and the shifts in fluid and some of the swelling that occurs around swollen joints and in the skin that we typically recognize as inflammation. These symptoms are all indicators that the immune system is attacking and ingesting the antigens. For example, the rash on the cheeks typical in lupus patients, called the *malar rash,* is the effect of these inflammatory mediators.

Can you explain the inflammation process in a little more detail?

Inflammation is caused by any insult or injury to a tissue or to a cell. The injury could be caused by pressure, trauma, heat, cold, an organism—whatever. It sets off an alarm, which activates a variety of cells. The cells come from the immune system and the bone marrow.

The immune system cells are the lymphocytes and the macrophages. The macrophage is the most important cell in this process. As antigen-presenting cells, the macrophages "register" the injury and determine if there is any foreign material at the site of the injury. When the macrophages determine that the material is foreign, they transmit a chemical code to the lymphocytes saying that this is a foreign invader and give detailed information about the invader, such as how many amino acids it has, what it looks like, and whether it's a fat, a sugar, a protein, and so on. It gives the immune system the memory to recognize this invader when it enters the body again.

The bone marrow cells are leukocytes. They come along and scoop up the foreign materials or the debris caused by the injury. These are the inflammatory cells. They come to the scene and release chemicals that cause swelling, inflammation, and pain. The area is walled off. It's flooded with fluids. And all of that inflammation, that pain, that swelling, and that fluid goes away when everything is cleaned up.

Why is there redness and pain with inflammation?

It is likely to be nature's way of protecting the area. It prevents you from further damaging the area that is already inflamed and painful. Your tendency is to not feel, rub, touch, or do anything to the area that is inflamed. Inflammation walls the area off from normal cells. An analogy would be putting yellow tape around a crime scene. It's to surround the area, to block off blood vessels. This blocking of the blood vessels causes the area to get red and painful.

The pain is, as far as the body is concerned, a minor aspect. It plays no essential role in clearing the damage. The pain is strictly for the organism's brain to prevent the organism from playing around, touching, rubbing, licking, or doing whatever else it might do to the area that might impede the healing process.

What are some of the chemicals involved in inflammation?

Prostaglandins and leukotrienes produce pain and swelling in various areas of the body and account for the migration of cells to an inflamed area. Drugs, such as aspirin, used to control the inflammatory response directly affect these chemicals in order to decrease inflammation.

The *prostaglandins* are a family of biologically active fats that are formed as a result of the action of an enzyme commonly known as a cyclooxygenase, or COX (see drug therapy on page 176). The most important action of the prostaglandins is the regulation of the inflammatory response.

The *leukotrienes* are another group of chemicals that do a number of things during the inflammatory response. Among the functions of the leukotrienes is their ability to bring white cells to an inflamed area and to increase the permeability of blood vessels, which accounts for swelling and redness.

What is pus?

Pus is nothing more than dead white cells—cells that have come to the area and participated in the inflammatory/destruction process.

Where does inflammation occur?

Inflammation can occur anywhere in the body. Most commonly, however, it occurs in joint spaces and other areas where there are white cells and immune complexes. Almost any organ can become inflamed.

What is collagen, and what role does it play in lupus?

Collagen is a complex molecule that makes up the "tough" areas or tissues of the body. It is strong enough to prevent a low-caliber bullet from cleanly exiting a human body. Skin consists, in part, of collagen, as do tendons, and the connections of muscles to bones. Collagen plays a very small role in lupus. Patients rarely make natural antibodies to collagen. That is why the old term "collagen disease," another term some people used for mixed connective tissue disease, is not accurate.

Why don't antibodies act the right way in people with lupus?

Antibodies are not the problem in lupus patients. The way the immune system incorrectly recognizes the self-substance as foreign is the problem. The antibodies do their jobs by attacking what the immune system tells them is a foreign substance.

TYPES OF LUPUS

What are some other names for lupus?

The disease is sometimes referred to as *systemic lupus erythematosus, SLE, LE,* or just plain *lupus. Systemic lupus erythematosus* is the proper medical term. Broken down, *systemic* means "all over" and *erythematosus* is "red."

How many different types of lupus are there?

There are three forms of lupus—*systemic lupus,* sometimes called *idiopathic lupus* or lupus of natural occurrence; *discoid lupus;* and *drug-induced lupus.*

What is the difference between them?

Systemic lupus is a more generalized disease, affecting virtually any body system, and is of unknown cause. *Discoid lupus* is basically lupus of the skin and also has no known cause. *Drug-induced lupus* is caused by specific ingested chemicals, such as medicines. It has been suggested that certain dietary factors (such as certain chemicals in one's diet that might be influencing immune function) may, like drugs, be among the causes of lupus; however, this has never been shown to be the case.

What is subacute cutaneous lupus?

Subacute cutaneous lupus is a particular form of systemic lupus that has characteristic skin changes. These changes in the skin can be very painful and itchy at the same time. This disease manifestation is somewhat difficult to control. A number of agents like cortisone, hydroxychloroquine, or Atabrine are used to control the symptoms. This condition is often associated with anti-Ro antibody and sometimes deficiencies of the early components of complement.

Discoid Lupus

What is discoid lupus?

Discoid lupus is lupus of the skin only. It can be a manifestation of systemic lupus, although it more often occurs by itself.

What are the symptoms of discoid lupus?

Discoid lupus can occasionally begin with symptoms that are not noticeable if they occur on the scalp or other place that's not visible or obvious. Discoid lupus usually begins in a patch of skin, which may change color or become red and scaly. Sometimes the skin becomes itchy as well. There can be hair loss when it occurs on the scalp or other hairy parts of the body. Scarring can occur in some cases. (The degree of scarring, as well as whether or not there are any permanent marks, varies from patient to patient.) Patients often mistake discoid lupus for a fungus or another less serious ailment.

How bad can discoid lupus get?

Generally a slowly progressing disease, discoid lupus can really worsen over time. Sun exposure or some substance such as a perfume or shampoo can make it worse. This form of lupus can cause extensive scarring and depigmentation (loss of pigmentation) in some areas. When these lesions get bigger and join together, they can be very disfiguring. The lesions are usually painless and, depending on the patient, can itch and become reddened.

How is discoid lupus diagnosed?

Discoid lupus can be accurately diagnosed with a biopsy of the skin. Sometimes physicians diagnose the disease without a skin biopsy because they are able to recognize its typical appearance. Other times, however, discoid lupus can be deceptive and less easy to detect. The diagnosis rests on the presence of immune complexes. In addition, after special preparation, when a piece of skin is examined under a particular type of microscope, a part of the skin called the *dermal-epidermal junction* "lights up" and is a fairly accurate indicator of the disease.

How is discoid lupus treated?

Discoid lupus can be treated in several ways. Local steroid creams or ointments can be used, or a steroid can be injected into the base of the lesion itself. In other cases, antimalarial drugs have been proved to be effective, although it is not known why they are helpful.

Are there specific steroids that can treat discoid lupus?

Many topical steroids can be used to treat discoid lupus. Different strengths of steroids can be used, depending on the location of the lesion. This is because stronger steroids applied as gels or ointments may cause shrinkage of the skin. When applied on the face or other sensitive parts of the body, this could be disfiguring.

Some topical corticosteroids include Diprolene (high potency), Topicort (high to medium potency, depending on the preparation), Lidex (high potency), Synalar (medium potency), Hydrocort, and Hytone (low potency). Most of these agents can be found as a cream, ointment, or gel base. Either your doctor or pharmacist can suggest the appropriate vehicle for application. Agents are used on different areas of the body, for example Hytone is used on the face and Diprolene is used on the arms or legs.

What are some of the antimalarials that can be used to treat discoid disease?

Some of the antimalarial drugs that can treat discoid disease include hydroxychloroquine and chloroquine. These are given at different doses and vary in strength. The precautions, namely an eye exam every six months because of eye toxicity in some people, are the same for both agents.

Are there methods to cover the depigmented areas on my skin?

There are various pigments and cosmetic products that can be purchased to protect and cover the depigmented areas of the skin. Many products such as Covermark are thicker than standard makeup and made hypoallergenic to avoid irritation of the skin. Standard makeup may be adequate depending on the degree of depigmentation and scarring.

How likely is it that discoid lupus will develop into SLE?

Not too likely, but it does happen in 10 to 15 percent of all cases. It is often assumed, incorrectly, that the skin lesions are a prelude to the systemic disease. Some people with discoid lupus inevitably have antibodies in their blood. But this means very little unless the person also has other signs and symptoms that suggest systemic lupus. Many doctors feel that discoid lupus patients might have some low-grade systemic symptoms. In these cases, the discoid lesions may be the first signs of systemic disease and, although it is rare, such individuals might go on to develop a more serious form of the disease.

Drug-Induced Lupus

Q What, exactly, happens in drug–
    induced lupus?

Drug-induced lupus comes on rather suddenly in a small number of
people taking certain drugs. This disease can mimic the natural disease.
No one knows just how it comes about, but the symptoms of lupus are
just as common in this form of the disease as they are in naturally occurring lupus.

Q What drugs are guilty of inducing
    lupus reactions?

The top three drugs are Pronestyl (procainamide), Apresoline (hydralazine), and INH (isoniazid). These drugs are used today with great
frequency. Procainamide is used to treat heart irregularities called arrhyth-
mias. Since most heart irregularities occur in men, men seem to make
up a large percentage of cases of drug-induced lupus. Hydralazine is
used to treat high blood pressure, and isoniazid is given for tuberculosis.
Since tuberculosis seems to be on the rise these days, the number of
INH-induced lupus cases is also on the rise. Other drugs that may cause
drug-induced lupus include beta blockers, tricyclic antidepressants, penicillin, and sulfa drugs.

Q Why do these drugs lead to drug–
    induced lupus?

No one really knows the cause, or mechanisms, of drug-induced lupus.
Old theories stated that the drugs would bind to DNA (deoxyribonu-
cleic acid) and create a new antigen, which would then become *immu-
nogenic* (capable of causing an immune reaction). However, this was proved

wrong. One recent theory is that these drugs activate the immune system in some unknown way. Another theory is that cumulative doses may play a role, but this would depend on the drug and the person. Drug-induced lupus is not an allergy. Interestingly, if you already have lupus, taking these drugs will not cause a flare of the disease.

Does one have to have a predisposition to drug-induced lupus, or could this happen to a normal, healthy person?

Drug-induced lupus does seem to depend on genetics. There are certain markers on cells that are thought to predispose people to certain diseases. These are called the *transplantation antigens* or *histocompatibility markers* (sort of like zip codes for cells). Most scientists believe that no disease can be acquired unless you have the appropriate genetic markers. One particular marker, DR4, has been linked to patients who get drug-induced disease, particularly those with hydralazine-induced lupus. Basically, however, the disease can be caused in anyone who takes medication and has the right biochemical and genetic makeup.

Systemic Lupus

What is systemic lupus?

Systemic lupus is a multiorgan disease of unknown cause that results in inflammation and dysfunction of one or many organs of the body.

Why is lupus referred to as systemic?

Because lupus can involve virtually every organ system of the body, the term *systemic,* meaning "general," is used to describe it. The rest of this book is devoted to providing much more information about systemic lupus.

THE INCIDENCE OF LUPUS

How common is lupus?

This depends on the ethnic and racial composition of a population. Lupus occurs more often in certain ethnic groups. The Caucasian incidence is roughly 1:1,000 (one person in every thousand). In African Americans, the numbers are higher (1:250); and in Latinos, the numbers are 1:500. There are also certain countries where the disease is quite common, such as China, Cambodia, and Thailand. Unfortunately, there are no statistics for the incidence of lupus in Asian Americans.

Why do different races have different rates?

No one knows why. The underlying reason for certain racial prevalence probably depends on genetic makeup.

Is it true that African-American women have more serious lupus?

Yes, it appears that African-American women have much more active lupus than other ethnic groups. In fact, the complications from severe kidney disease are greater in the African-American community. The reasons for this difference in activity do not seem to depend on socio-economic factors; however, the most severe manifestations are usually worse in people who wait to have their disease diagnosed or who have poor access to competent physicians.

Do the people of Africa have the same instance of lupus as African Americans?

It appears that lupus is less common in Africa, although the lower numbers may reflect the fact that accurate numbers are not available. A variety of studies reveal that lupus in the African patient is just as severe as that found in African Americans. There may be other factors involved in the reported lower incidence of overall autoimmunity.

Is lupus considered to be a rare disease?

No. If one calculates the numbers in this country, the prevalence is high—approximately 500,000 people or more by currently accepted studies. However, most estimates are based on hospitalized patients, whereas the great majority of patients who are diagnosed are not hospitalized. Recently, organizations like the Lupus Foundation of American have investigated the issue and estimated the numbers of people who say they have been diagnosed with lupus in America to be anywhere from 2 to 2.5 million.

The number of people with lupus worldwide is not known. Only time and future scientific studies will provide a true picture.

Are the number of cases of lupus on the rise?

It would seem so. However, this may be due to the improved ability to diagnose the disease. It might also be due to the fact that many people who have autoantibodies but do not meet the other criteria of the disease are diagnosed (possibly incorrectly) as lupus patients.

What are some other reasons for this apparent increase?

There is more awareness of lupus because of organizations like the Lupus Foundation of America. Physicians also have better access to laboratories that specialize in immunological testing.

Is there a particular age at which lupus begins to affect a person?

The most common ages for the onset of lupus are between the ages of 18 and 55. Some can be diagnosed at earlier ages, even in early childhood. There are also many cases of lupus occurring in old age, particularly in men. Regardless of the age at which lupus begins, it lasts for the rest of the person's life. It is the age of onset that varies.

Can one get lupus after 50?

For reasons that are not clear, lupus can occur for the first time at a later age. Some researchers suggest that this could be due to some change in thyroid function or, as is the case with men, a drop in the level of male hormones. It is now clear that women who have active lupus will have a decrease of clinical activity after the menopause or change of life.

How many new cases are diagnosed each year?

Roughly 16,000.

Do women get lupus more often than men?

Far more women get lupus than men, primarily during the childbearing years. The ratio is currently estimated to be one man with lupus for every ten to fifteen women. An interesting fact that is the focus of much research is that before puberty (1:3) and after menopause (1:8) the disease affects men and women more equally than the 1:10–15 ratio.

Why is lupus more prevalent in women?

The reasons are not clear. What is clear is that female hormones affect the severity of the disease. Estrogen does not cause the disease, but estrogens can have an effect on the strength of the antibodies that appear. This hormone might even contribute to certain cytokine profiles that enhance immune activity and be responsible for symptoms such as joint pains and fever.

Does lupus manifest itself differently in men versus women?

Lupus's effects vary between the sexes and from person to person. Some studies suggest that lupus can affect men more severely than women. However, the vast majority of clinicians will tell you that men tend to have milder forms of the disease. Active female hormones tend to stimulate the immune system and consequently make female lupus patients feel worse. No one really knows exactly how these hormones affect the immune system. Some researchers say that they stimulate the cells to make more antibody, while others say the immune system cells are "boosted" by the hormones.

CAUSES OF LUPUS

What causes lupus?

It is still not known what causes lupus. Research is ongoing to investigate both the *causes* of lupus (what is responsible for lupus existing in the first place) and the *triggers* of a lupus flare (what is responsible for bringing out the symptoms of the disease).

What is the difference between a cause and a trigger?

It is important to distinguish between these two terms. For lupus to become evident, there has to be both a cause and a trigger, but the terms have different meanings. The cause of lupus (which is still unknown) is what created the potential for the person to have the disease. The trigger is what brings out the symptoms of lupus—a factor or circumstance that causes the disease to manifest itself in evident signs and symptoms. In other words, the trigger is the specific factor or factors that cause a flare of the disease. Some people may incorrectly use these terms interchangeably.

There are factors that are associated with, but do not cause, lupus. These often include gender (female) and perhaps some association of certain histocompatibility genes, or those genes responsible for the immune response.

Many women have what is called a *lupus diathesis,* which is essentially a tendency to acquire lupus. Many autoimmune diseases that are not lupus come forward after a viral infection or some other provocative factor that boosts the immune system. These patients are often called patients with incomplete lupus or those having a lupus diathesis.

So there isn't one currently accepted theory of the cause of lupus?

No. Lupus is multifactorial. In other words, it depends on so many factors that it is hard to pinpoint one specific cause. Most scientists believe that the cause is a combination of genetic susceptibility and environmental factors.

The disease closely resembles the syndrome of a chronic infection. That is why it is the belief of many clinicians and investigators that lupus is really an infectious disease that occurs as a result of some unusual virus or other undetermined agent.

There are many theories about the causes of lupus. One theory is defective suppressor cell function. This theory is based on the idea that the immune system is normally held in "check" by cells that prevent it from overacting. These are called *suppressor cells.* Although not likely to be the exact cause of the disease, these cells are certainly involved in the disease process.

Another more current and popular theory is that a gene in some mammals (specifically the mouse, where this was described), called the *fas* gene, is defective. This is important as an idea since we have found many genes to be like the fas gene, and it is possible that more might eventually be discovered.

A hypothesis for humans, based on mouse research, is that when the immune system develops, certain cells show *autoreactivity*—that is, they react with one's own cells and tissues. These cells are naturally destroyed by Mother Nature before birth. There are genes in the body that know of the autoreactive cells, and they program other cells to destroy them. It is the fas gene that regulates this process of cell death, called *apoptosis.* The theory is that there are times that the fas gene becomes defective and does not do its job to regulate necessary cell death. When that happens, the autoreactive cells continue to live and are responsible for increased autoreactive activity. This may result in an autoimmune disease such as lupus. This provides an interesting area for research—to find out why this gene does become defective and if anything can possibly be done to change it using gene therapy.

How can lupus be treated without knowing its cause?

Lupus patients all share similar symptoms based on inflammatory processes. Fever, weakness, aches, and pains are all common aspects of this unique disease. We do know how to treat these various symptom complexes. In essence, it is the symptoms that are being treated and not the real disease, since the actual cause is still unknown.

Hormones as a Factor

What research is currently ongoing regarding gender and lupus?

Although lupus is called a disease of the childbearing years, men also acquire the illness. Older women and young children can get the disease too. Research currently revolves around the female reproductive system simply because removal of the ovaries and uterus has resulted in significant improvement in laboratory animals. This observation was first made in animals and then in humans. This is not intended to suggest that hysterectomies are the cure for lupus. But a woman who requires a hysterectomy due to other medical problems may see an improvement in her lupus.

As is often the case with research, discoveries come with more frequency when two different disciplines—such as endocrinology, the study of the endocrine system and the treatment of its problems, and rheumatology, the study and treatment of rheumatic conditions or diseases of connective tissue and joints—share essential information.

What exactly are hormones?

Hormones are small molecules that regulate all sorts of bodily functions. They are the chemicals that are responsible for secondary sexual characteristics, such as hair on the face or the size of one's breasts. In a woman, the major hormones are the *estrogens*. They are produced by the ovaries before menopause and by the adrenal glands after. Men produce hormones called *androgens* in their testicles. Men produce very little estrogen, and women produce very little androgen. However, it is important to note that both sexes produce both kinds of hormone. Evidence indicates that these hormones are potent regulators of immune function and, consequently, have an effect on lupus.

How do hormones affect lupus?

Hormones can have either a good or bad effect on lupus in animals. In humans, their effects are not clear. Estrogens generally stimulate the immune system, whereas the reverse is true of androgens (male hormones). Research has not shown that men and women with lupus produce abnormal levels of hormones. However, there may be certain metabolic abnormalities in people with lupus. *Metabolism* is the process of conversion of one chemical to another. Women with lupus, according to some studies, may have a more rapid metabolism of male hormones. In addition, estrogen can be rapidly converted to various inactive or active *metabolites,* products of metabolism, in both men and women with SLE. This can make lupus worse or better, depending on whether there is an excess or deficiency of certain metabolites.

Do hormones have anything to do with lupus?

The *pituitary gland* is a small gland located in the center of the brain that produces the "master" hormones that affect the other glands of the body, such as the testicles and the ovaries, the thyroid, and the adrenal glands. Hormones such as prolactin and the sex hormones have major roles in immune system function and are thought to have an association with lupus.

How does prolactin affect lupus?

Prolactin is the hormone from the pituitary gland that causes the production of mother's milk. If a woman has tenderness of the breasts all the time and secretion of milk when she is not pregnant or nursing, it could suggest elevated prolactin levels. High levels of prolactin are stimulatory to the immune system, and instances of high prolactin levels have been found in both men and women with lupus and related diseases like anemia. In animals, injection of prolactin or transplantation of extra pituitary cells can cause a condition similar to lupus. If a woman with both lupus and tender breasts has elevated prolactin, then the pro-lactin levels and possibly the lupus can be treated with bromocriptine, an antiprolactin drug. It is common practice in some countries to give prolactin inhibitors to patients with active lupus. However, there are many studies that do not support the idea that prolactin is involved in the cause of lupus.

How do sex hormones affect lupus?

It is clear that sex hormones play a major role in the regulation of the immune system. It appears that estrogen activates the immune system and can make a disease like lupus more severe. Conversely, male sex hormones may have the reverse effect.

Should women with lupus take birth control pills?

Birth control pills, which contain estrogen and sometimes progesterone, are not advised for women with lupus, particularly those who have a propensity for clotting, as estrogens enhance this clotting. Research on the effects of birth control pills on lupus is still pending, and the risks have not fully been evaluated.

Can a woman with lupus take hormone replacement therapy?

Hormone replacement therapy (HRT) is a hormone therapy involving some form of estrogen taken after menopause begins; HRT is taken to prevent osteoporosis, hot flashes, and other symptoms of menopause. Today, however, there is much controversy about the relation between the ingestion of hormone replacement therapy and the risk of conditions such as Alzheimer's disease and various cancers.

The good news is that anecdotal evidence suggests that HRT can be taken if the dose of estrogen is not above levels that would normally occur in the body and if the clinical activity of the patient's disease is monitored by her physician. The risks of taking hormone replacement therapy include things like phlebitis and clot formation in the legs. Lupus patients who have "sticky blood" antibodies are at greater risk for developing these clots on this medication. Studies are being conducted to evaluate the safety of taking HRT in patients with lupus. A study called the Selena trial has just been finished. This study is designed to look at the safety of oral contraceptives use and HRT in women with lupus. Hopefully, this study will tell us about the safety of these hormones in lupus.

Is there anything that would absolutely preclude my taking any sex hormone?

Yes, any propensity for clotting precludes you from taking any hormones. Hormones are also not to be taken by patients who smoke or have a history of vascular disease.

Heredity as a Factor

Is lupus inherited?

There is no question that lupus can be inherited in some manner, although lupus is not considered a genetic disease in the classical sense. Relatives of lupus patients have an approximately 5 to 12 percent greater tendency to get the disease if family members have it. We say that there may be a genetic predisposition to developing the disease. These family members generally have what are termed *immune response genes* that predispose them to the illness. The immune response genes can be identified, but this very lengthy process is not routinely available. Many people with the appropriate immune response genes have what is called a *relative risk* for the disease. This generally means that there are several factors that have to act, in addition to the presence of genes, in order for someone to actually contract the disease. Certain ethnic groups have higher relative risks than others.

What research is currently underway regarding the genetics of lupus?

There is a great deal of research at present. In fact, the human genome project, which has been underway for many years, revolves around the idea that knowledge of the entire human genome (a complete set of genes in the chromosomes from one parent) would be helpful in better understanding the genetic bases for a variety of diseases.

There are a total of forty-six chromosomes in the body. Chromosome 6 is where the immune response genes are located in humans. The immune response genes are involved in the process of presenting substances to cells. They determine whether or not one is susceptible to certain diseases. A fundamental question in lupus research is whether there is a constitutive gene that is not on chromosome 6 that can affect an individual's risk for getting SLE.

What about research that suggests that there is a problem gene on chromosome 1 in lupus patients?

Some very new data has been found from family studies to show that a gene on chromosome 1 is related to the acquisition of lupus. Over fifty families were studied. The significance of this finding is not known at present. However, the inspiration for this discovery came from studies in certain lupus mice where chromosome 1 has always been involved in the acquisition of the disease. It seems that the same findings could apply to humans with lupus.

How do familial studies help in understanding the genetics of lupus?

Familial studies allow careful analysis of inherited genes, of which immune response genes are present in the affected versus the unaffected family member, and of the correlation between lupus and other genetic factors, such as gender. Within a family, studies are particularly useful if more than one family member is affected and, more important, if more than one generation is affected. Unfortunately for researchers, in SLE, an immune response gene can be present but the patient may not have the disease. Again, the disease is multifactorial.

What is the role of twins in this study?

Twins offer some opportunities for interesting study. This is particularly true of identical twins, who also have identical genetics. Even in identical twins in which one has lupus, the disease will only occur in the other identical twin approximately 25 percent of the time. This indicates that even if your chromosomes are identical to those of someone with lupus, you will not necessarily get it. Despite extensive studies of twins, more research is necessary to figure out why and how lupus occurs in those with the appropriate immune response genes.

Can a person develop lupus if there is no family history of the illness?

Absolutely! These sporadic occurrences of lupus are particularly difficult to understand. It is likely, however, that there are other diseases in the family that are related to lupus or have some bearing on the disease. These are usually other autoimmune diseases like *Sjogren's syndrome* (an autoimmune disease characterized by autoimmune reactions to glands such as the salivary and tear glands, resulting in a lack of tears, saliva, and other glandular secretions), rheumatoid arthritis, low platelet disorders, or various kinds of anemia. If curious, a patient can look into his or her family history to try to uncover various known abnormalities.

Other Possible Factors

What other causal theories are being investigated?

Other causal theories of lupus include dietary and environmental causes; however, these theories have not yet been thoroughly researched and proven. Unusual (and stealthy) bacterial organisms such as *mycoplasmas* and *retroviruses* might also be causes yet to be identified.

What are mycoplasmas?

Mycoplasmas are thought by many to be bacteria that have no cell walls. As a result, they just sort of meld into the background. For years it has been thought that they may be involved in the cause of arthritis. (They do cause arthritis in rats and mice!) In people, we have never been able to isolate mycoplasmas as the cause of rheumatoid arthritis or lupus. One reason for this is that the methods to grow mycoplasmas are so crude and difficult that, even though they could be the cause of disease, they are virtually undetectable.

What are retroviruses?

Retroviruses were unknown until two decades ago. To understand why retroviruses are being studied, we need to introduce the function of DNA, which is literally the building block of life. DNA, genes, and chromosomes are involved in the process of the reproduction of life and are the mechanisms by which changes in cells can occur. DNA molecules are found mainly in the chromosomes inside cell nuclei, which are the carriers of genetic information. DNA is the "template," the master

pattern from which cells make *ribonucleic acid* (RNA). Similar in structure and composition to DNA, RNA then uses the genetic instructions
received from the DNA to create proteins in all living cells.

Most viruses prefer to use DNA as a means of replication. There are
some viruses, however, that use RNA as the genetic material template
for reproduction, instead of DNA. They then transmit the instructions
backward (retro) to the DNA. Because these retroviruses can cause
problems for the cell's genetic activities, research is exploring the possible connection between this and the immune dysfunction involved in
lupus.

Viruses are often very difficult to detect and isolate. Retroviruses are
even more difficult to detect and isolate than regular DNA-replicated
viruses. Because of their ability to avoid detection, it is possible that
these viruses could hide until the appropriate stimulus comes along to
make them active again. It was believed, and still is, that because these
viruses are so difficult to find and replicate in the laboratory, maybe this
is one of the causes of lupus.

Can lupus be sexually transmitted?

Lupus cannot be sexually transmitted, although there are numerous reports of spouses of lupus patients developing autoantibodies. However,
this is believed to occur by chance and is unlikely to be significant.

LUPUS AND ITS RELATION TO OTHER DISEASES

Why is lupus call "the great imitator"?

Over the centuries, several of the more complicated diseases, such as diabetes and syphilis, have been called "great imitators." Lupus, a multi-
systemic illness, has also acquired this label because it can mimic other
diseases.

What diseases are most similar to lupus?

Many rheumatic diseases (characterized by stiff muscles and/or sore joints) are similar to lupus. The closest are Sjogren's syndrome and rheumatoid arthritis. Blood disorders like anemias, clotting deficiencies, diseases of the *platelets* (blood cell fragments that play a critical role in the clotting of blood and wound repair), and disorders of white cells also resemble lupus. Lupus can be mimicked by kidney diseases caused by an illness, such as diabetes. Various skin rashes can resemble lupus, such as those found in the *pemphigoid* diseases (autoimmune skin illnesses). Many neurological, pulmonary, cardiac, and musculoskeletal diseases can mimic lupus. Lyme disease and other less specific diseases such as chronic fatigue syndrome may also be confused with lupus.

What are some of the similarities between lupus and these other diseases?

Symptoms that lupus has in common with some of these other diseases include the presence of joint pain, antibodies, and rash. Fatigue, fever, and muscle aches are also common symptoms of these diseases.

What differentiates these diseases?

Sometimes it is very difficult to distinguish between lupus and these other diseases. Laboratory test results can either help or hinder a final diagnosis. For example, *rheumatoid arthritis* (RA) is considered by many to be a "cousin" of lupus, but it is very different. Both are autoimmune diseases, but rheumatoid arthritis has fewer autoimmune features than lupus. The major autoantibody that is measured in RA is the *rheumatoid factor,* or an antibody against other antibodies. The rheumatoid factors are very typical of rheumatoid arthritis, whereas the antibodies of the lupus patient are usually directed against specific antigens that are not other antibodies. Lupus patients usually do not have rheumatoid factors.

Clinically, the diseases are also very different. Rheumatoid arthritis is largely a symmetrical disease (each side of the body is affected in a similar manner—both knees hurt, both hips hurt, etc.) affecting a number of joints. It causes erosions in the bones of the hands, feet, and knee joints. Rheumatoid arthritis is a disease of the moveable joints that causes destruction of them. This is not the case with lupus.

Another related disease is *scleroderma,* a disease resulting in *sclerosis,* or hardening of tissue. The antibodies in scleroderma patients are usually directed toward *antitopoisomerase,* or DNA-unwinding protein. There is no abundance of autoantibody as seen in lupus. The main symptoms of this disease are also different. They include difficulty swallowing, malabsorption (inadequate absorption of nutrients into the intestines) due to thickening of the bowel wall, thickened skin, deep skin pigmentation, and thickening of blood vessels that can result in severe hypertension.

Dermatomyositis also presents itself differently. It is an autoimmune disease of muscle. The patient produces antibody against certain muscle enzymes (an *enzyme* is a protein that works as a catalyst for a specific function). Physical symptoms associated with this illness include so-called raccoon eyes, pain, and weakness of the muscles near the trunk (such as in the upper arms and thighs).

Can a person with lupus get another autoimmune disease?

Yes. This is not uncommon. Antibodies can develop against a variety of organs, tissues, or glands, resulting in many different diseases. For example, a person with lupus can have *Hashimoto's thyroiditis,* in which antibodies can be made to the thyroid gland. On the other hand, Hashimoto's thyroiditis may occur by itself in patients. It doesn't need to occur with lupus. Any autoantibodies can occur in and of themselves, or as part of lupus. However, once a patient has lupus, all related autoimmune phenomena are usually considered to be under the umbrella of lupus.

What are common autoimmune diseases that may be diagnosed in somebody who has already been diagnosed with lupus?

Among the diseases lupus patients most frequently experience are Sjo-gren's syndrome, multiple sclerosis, Hashimoto's thyroiditis, autoimmune liver disease, and a very rare condition called porphyria. Fibromyalgia, chronic fatigue syndrome, and conditions such as antiphospholipid syn-drome (see page 149) are common to lupus patients. It is important to understand that almost any other autoimmune disease can exist in a pa-tient with lupus erythematosus.

Can a lupus patient be diagnosed with rheumatoid arthritis?

It is unusual to have rheumatoid arthritis and lupus at the same time, al-though some people believe it does happen. There are others who think that there is a condition called "rhupus," which is a combination of the two diseases. Lupus and rheumatoid arthritis are closely related by auto-antibodies, hence the similarities bring about a lot of confusion.

THE COURSE OF LUPUS

Do all individuals with lupus have the same symptoms?

No. Symptoms vary from patient to patient. They even vary within one patient from time to time. Since lupus is a disease that can attack differ-ent organ systems of the body, it affects everyone differently. Even in ge-netically identical twins, the presentation of lupus usually isn't the same.

Can an individual with lupus continue to develop new symptoms?

Generally, a patient's symptoms may vary from week to week. However, it is uncommon for the affected organ system to change. For example, it is rare for a patient with kidney disease to develop central nervous system lupus or lung lupus as a new symptom.

Do people with lupus get sick often?

Unfortunately, individuals with lupus do tend to get sick quite often. Some patients get sick cyclically. For example, some experts note that most patients are sickest in the winter months, particularly December. Changes in the seasons are also associated with a great number of lupus flares.

Without careful management by a qualified specialist, this disease can take on many forms and be quite troublesome. However, quality clinical care can improve the patient's overall quality of life.

When might a person with lupus have to go to the hospital?

As with other diseases, patients with lupus must be hospitalized if their disease becomes life-threatening. Patients are also admitted at the start of any kind of serious treatment. Other problems that might require hospitalization include serious bleeding, low platelets, kidney failure with nausea and vomiting, hypotension or low blood pressure, or an inability to breathe due to fluid in the lungs.

What is the normal course of lupus?

The normal course of lupus is unpredictable. There are periods of complete remission that are coupled with periods of disease activity called flares. A *flare* is a time when a lupus patient becomes sick for a period of time. While there are many factors that can affect the course of the disease and produce flares, most are not known. It is known that stress, illness, and overall exhaustion can make the disease worse and can cause a flare. The average lupus patient can have as little as one and as many as six flares per year. The object of treating the patient is to prevent flares that are immune rejections of his or her own cells and tissues. If lupus is left untreated, death can result.

What is the course of lupus in children?

Some clinicians believe that the disease may be worse in children than in adults. Others disagree. However, childhood lupus can become very active at puberty, when the hormones are very active.

Flares and Remissions

What is a flare?

A *flare* is a sudden change of disease activity, for example, the development of new symptoms. A patient may suddenly feel weak, run a low temperature, have joint and muscle aches, and develop oral and nasal ulcers. Flares can take on many different forms, indicating that the disease is quite active.

What is an exacerbation?

An *exacerbation* is a "worsening" and is a term that is generally synonymous with a flare.

How long do flares last?

Untreated, a flare can last for days, even weeks. The disease can gradually worsen, and the patient may get very sick. However, a flare can often be abruptly terminated with immunosuppressive medications, such as prednisone.

Does everybody experience a flare in the same way?

Flares are experienced differently by different people.

What can the individual do to prevent flares?

Routine checkups are a good start, especially in times of severe stress or at those times of the year when the disease seems to worsen. Keep stress to a minimum. Wear sunblock to prevent exposure to the sun. Rest. Avoid overexertion. Although there may be things you can do to reduce the chances of flares, they often occur regardless of any preventive efforts made. It is not totally within your power to control flares, but you can consult your doctor and get specific blood tests in order to avoid a major flare. A great deal of research is dedicated to the prediction of lupus flares.

What is remission?

A *remission* is a period when you are disease-free. Certain cases of lupus have become permanently inactive, or in *total remission*. Although total remission is rare, partial remission—a definite, but limited, period of inactive disease—is more common.

How many people go into remission?

Almost all patients with lupus go into remission at one time or another. This depends largely on the skill of the physician. Partial remission is possible with proper medication and attitude and periods of rest.

How often does remission occur?

A remission can occur any number of times during the year. As patients become more adept at managing their diseases with medication and behavioral changes, the periods of time between periods of remission can lengthen.

How long do remissions last?

Partial remissions can last a long time. Some patients may have no lupus activity for six months to a year, while others may experience remission for only a few weeks. Total remission can last a lifetime—although laboratory tests may remain positive, the actual clinical disease can become inactive.

How many flares can one have per year?

The average lupus patient has from one to six flares per year.

What are some of the indicators of disease exacerbation my doctor should look for?

Most of the following must be confirmed by your doctor since some or many of these could be chronically present in many patients:

- Fatigue
- Fever
- Rash
    - Rash on the cheeks
    - A raised rash with little white bumps
    - Redness of fingertips, tips of toes, areas around fingernails, or the palms or the soles of the feet
    - Areas of *vasculitis* (inflammation of small blood vessels), which could be characterized by small ulcers
    - Fishnet pattern to the skin
    - Fluid- or air-filled blisters
    - Deep pockets of inflamed and sometimes ulcerated skin
- Loss of hair
- Sun sensitivity
- Ulcers in the mouth or nose
- Joint pains
- Small nodules on the tendons (around the elbow or on the ankles)
- Muscle inflammation
- Enlarged lymph nodes
- Enlargement of the parotid glands (the glands in the cheeks)
- Inflammation of the lining of the lungs or the heart
- Low platelet count
- Low white count or low lymphocyte count
- High blood pressure
- Menstrual period irregularities
- Sore throat, backache, or headache
- Eye problems
    - Spots in the eyes called "cotton wool spots" and sometimes little hemorrhages
    - Little clotted blood vessels in the eyes (found by your doctor)

- Abnormalities of complement (low complement or absence of one component of the complement pathway)
- Antibodies to *cardiolipin* (a substance obtained from the heart muscle of a cow that is used as an antigen in tests for syphilis and lupus)
- The *lupus anticoagulant* (antibodies that are usually directed against platelets or certain clotting factors, but conversely, in lupus, are dangerous because they actually encourage clotting to occur)

What are some of the indicators that could suggest other lupus-related diseases?

It is important for your physician to clearly delineate the symptoms of lupus-related autoimmune diseases. Some of the most common indicators that could suggest other autoimmune diseases include:

- Severe muscle pain, indicating an immune-mediated muscle disease such as polymyositis or the muscle inflammation of lupus or fibromyalgia; your doctor can tell if the pain is from muscle inflammation
- An enlarged painful thyroid, indicating Graves' disease or Hashimoto's thyroiditis
- Dry eyes and mouth along with large parotid glands (the glands in the cheeks), indicating secondary Sjogren's syndrome

Numbness, tingling, and loss of balance could mean involvement of the nervous system.

TRIGGERS OF LUPUS FLARES

What can trigger a lupus flare?

There are many possible triggers of a lupus flare. These can be divided into two categories: *endogenous* (inner) and *exogenous* (external). Endogenous triggers include a cold, physical stress, exhaustion, a viral illness, or injury. Exogenous triggers include sunlight, fluorescent light, or emotional stressors such as divorce, illness, or death in the family. Other possibilities, which have not yet been scientifically confirmed as triggers, include dietary indiscretions, such as high-fat diets, or environmental factors, such as X-rays and microwaves.

Are triggers always easy to identify?

No, since it is not always known what may cause a flare.

Can excessive fatigue trigger a flare?

Yes. There is a correlation between what goes on in the brain and lupus activity. One form of significant stress is fatigue. Therefore, it can certainly cause a flare of the disease.

Can lack of sleep (three or four hours a night for example) be a cause of lupus?

No. However, when a predisposition to autoimmune disease is present, excessive fatigue can trigger the onset of the disease. There may be a propensity toward lupus, or the presence of antibodies that were never previously detected. These can become apparent at this time. But because lack of sleep or rest can trigger a worsening of the disease, one of our first therapeutic suggestions is to get enough rest.

How does sunlight trigger a flare?

No one really understands the effect of sunlight on lupus. Moreover, some people with lupus can be exposed to sun with no unusual effects.

What is the role of anxiety or other emotional factors in triggering a lupus flare?

Stress is a factor that has been associated with lupus flares. The intimate connections between a person's brain and the immune system are not yet fully understood. Perhaps stress on one system results in stress on a similar, yet different, system, namely the immune system.

What is the connection between allergies and lupus?

An allergic state produces a very specific antibody to exogenous substances like drugs, pollen, and grass. People with lupus are often hypersensitive to such agents. For example, lupus patients may be particularly sensitive to sulfa drugs (drugs containing sulfur) and are told to stay away from them. Curiously, many patients with lupus also pinpoint a specific antibiotic, like penicillin, as the trigger of a reaction.

What is the connection between hair dyes and lupus?

Hair dyes and colorings have been implicated as possible triggers of lupus flares in some people. This suspicion rests on the fact that the presence of certain dyes (hair coloring) is important to the development of some forms of drug-induced disease. However, recent data has indicated that there is no association between hair dyes and lupus.

Why might radiation therapy cause a flare?

Many radiation therapists clearly avoid radiation therapy in patients who have active disease. The theory behind this is that radiation causes the death of many cells in a particular site (the target site). When these cells die, internal contents of the cells are extruded, and the patient becomes immunized to his or her own cellular content. Since the patient already makes antibodies against certain proteins and other chemicals from within the cell, it is assumed that immunization with more cell content as the result of radiation will only cause a heightened immune response and, therefore, a worsening of the lupus.

OTHER COMMON QUESTIONS

Is lupus infectious or contagious?

Some people get confused about the difference between the meanings of *infectious* and *contagious*. *Infectious* means an organism, such as a virus or bacteria, has infected the person. On the other hand, *contagious* means that something is transmissible or communicable—such as a disease that can be "caught" by, or transmitted to, another person. If something is infectious, that does not mean that it is contagious (although in some cases it may be).

Most probably, lupus is not contagious. Scientists have not been able to identify a bacterium or virus that might be responsible for the disease. However, there have been reports of individuals developing autoantibodies after marriage to someone with lupus. At this point, however, it is believed that this is probably more coincidental than anything else. There is still no conclusive proof that lupus is contagious.

We cannot say at this time that lupus is infectious, or caused by a microorganism. Some experts are investigating the theory that an infectious agent that is not transmissible in a classical sense might be the ultimate cause of the disease, but no conclusive evidence has yet been found.

Is lupus a type of cancer?

No. While lupus is incurable, it is not terminal. *Cancer* is the unchecked multiplication and growth of cells in a part of the body, such as a gland

TRIGGERS OF LUPUS FLARES

· · · · · ·

There are many things that can trigger a lupus flare. Most of them are not known. However, the following list includes things that have been observed by several investigators as the cause of a lupus flare.

- *Sunlight.* No one really understands the effect of sunlight on lupus. But there's no question that sunlight can (and does) cause flares in many (35 to 50 percent or more) patients with the disease. On the other hand, some people with lupus can be exposed to sun with no unusual effects.
- *Ultraviolet light,* from the sun or even from fluorescent lamps, may also be detrimental to certain patients.
- *Infections* are always stressful events. Viral and bacterial infections can trigger lupus flares.
- *Stress* of many different varieties can cause a flare of lupus. Examples of stressors include the loss of a loved one, a disease in the family, or even the stress of an examination.
- *Surgical procedures* are inherently very stressful. Surgical procedures such as a gallbladder operation, replacement of a hip, or a bypass operation are all stressful enough to require careful observation.
- *Pregnancy/abortion.* Changes during pregnancy, the delivery of a baby, or an abortion can also trigger flares.
- *Sulfa drugs* (drugs that contain sulfur) may cause adverse reactions in patients with lupus. (This is not a universal rule, but it is so commonly observed it should be mentioned.)
- *Birth control pills* are usually estrogen-containing substances. Whether birth control pills cause exacerbation or worsening of lupus is very unclear at this time. The same is true for hormone replacement therapy after menopause.
- *Radiation therapy* is indeed a cause of flare in patients who have had surgery for cancer and also have lupus.

or an organ, that may spread to other parts of the body. In lupus patients, there is no abnormal growth of any kind of tissue. Sometimes the lymph nodes can be enlarged, leading physicians to suspect that their patient is suffering from a cancer of the lymph cells. Only after biopsy can one see that the cells of such lymph nodes are not malignant (cancerous) but simply "hyperactive."

Do patients with lupus have a higher risk of cancer?

There appears to be a higher incidence of breast malignancies and abnormal cervical cell abnormalities in patients with lupus. This topic has been debated over many years, and no clear conclusion about the incidence of cancer has been established.

Will my lupus be affected by my cancer treatment?

There is some discussion and literature about the dangers of radiation therapy in patients who have lupus. The belief by many radiation oncologists is that radiation treatment can make lupus active. Therefore, it is the practice of many radiation oncologists to not give radiation to patients who have lupus. Chemotherapy, on the other hand, seems to have a beneficial effect for lupus patients, since this is merely adding to, or replacing, therapies that have already been given to lupus patients.

Is lupus a type of AIDS?

No. AIDS patients lose their immune functions because their T cells are infected and destroyed. As a result, AIDS patients have an underactive immune system (*hypo*immune function), which is much less able to fight foreign invaders, making the body much more vulnerable. In lupus, the reverse is true. No lymphocytes are lost, and the immune system is overactive, or *hyper*active. In addition, the AIDS virus is an example of a virus in the retroviral family. There is, despite ongoing research being conducted in this area, no evidence yet of retroviral infection in lupus.

What is the prognosis for people with lupus?

In general, the prognosis for people with lupus is excellent. One's life-span should not be shortened because of lupus. The prognosis for a lupus patient, because of earlier diagnosis and more aggressive treatment (where necessary), has improved significantly over the past twenty years.

The major problem for people with lupus occurs when the disease affects a major organ system. This requires aggressive treatment, but, unless some major organ system is severely compromised, the disease can still usually be controlled.

What are some of the factors that may affect the prognosis?

Each case is different. Developing a prognosis in long-term disease depends on such factors as the drugs used to control the disease, overall activity of the illness, the organs affected, the patient's age and gender, and the results of laboratory testing. For example, someone with kidney failure will have a much worse prognosis than someone who has only difficult-to-treat skin disease.

What is the mortality rate for individuals with lupus?

Lupus patients have a very low mortality rate compared with the rate of ten years ago. A small minority of patients die today. This difference is probably due to the aggressive treatment of the disease and to earlier diagnosis.

The mortality rate varies with ethnic group and race. For example, one study in 1978 suggested that the highest mortality rates were for black women, who died at a rate of 18 per million per year. This was followed by white women (6 per million), black men (3 per million), and then white men (2 per million). These numbers, however, are not the same for all studies and continue to change. However, the order is consistent in all studies; in other words, the mortality rate is highest for black women and lowest for white men.

What is the life expectancy for a patient diagnosed with SLE in childhood?

The prognosis for someone developing lupus as a child may not be as good as for someone who develops the disease in adulthood. But, once again, the disease depends on many other variables.

For those people who do die of lupus, what's the cause of death?

The most common cause of death was once infection. Steroids and other immunosuppressive drugs used to control lupus make patients more vulnerable to infection, which can be dangerous. However, the patients who experienced dangerous effects from these drugs were usually not closely supervised by their doctors. These patients had white cell counts that dropped without their knowledge, they had some major unknown debilitation, or they had an adverse reaction to the drugs. These effects are not common if the patient is being cared for by a competent specialist who knows how to administer immunosuppressive drugs and what side effects to watch for. In addition, the discovery of many new antibiotics has virtually eliminated this cause of death for most lupus patients.

The most common cause of death in lupus patients today is cardiovascular disease. Lupus patients suffer from high blood pressure more often and have more heart attacks at a younger age than the normal population. There are many possible reasons for this, including disordered lipid metabolism (for example, high cholesterol), side effects of drugs used to treat the disease, and perhaps an immunological basis for atherosclerosis that is exaggerated in patients with lupus.

2.

DIAGNOSING LUPUS

. . . .

The diagnosis of lupus is not a simple process. There is no test designed specifically to detect lupus. Because the symptoms of lupus are so similar to those of other diseases, patients must undergo many tests, and many criteria must be met before a patient is diagnosed with lupus. Undoubtedly, you may find it difficult to understand what each of these tests was designed to determine. This chapter attempts to answer the many questions you may have regarding the steps taken in the diagnosis of lupus.

SOME GENERAL INFORMATION

How long does it take to diagnose lupus?

Although an astute physician may diagnose lupus fairly quickly, there have been cases where the disease has taken anywhere from five to ten years to be diagnosed. Some patients are never diagnosed. Of course, those that are able to escape diagnosis are usually the less severe cases of lupus.

The physician caring for lupus patients must be an expert on this disease. That is why it is so important to see a rheumatologist who has a fine working knowledge of lupus and its related maladies. It requires great effort to distinguish lupus from other diseases or to establish any overlap syndromes.

Can lupus be diagnosed in utero?

No. There are no genetic tests to predict the onset of lupus, and the mother's antibodies are present in a baby's blood for many months. Neonatal lupus does not mean that a baby will have lupus but merely that the mother's antibodies are present. These antibodies from the mother go away when the baby begins to make its own.

If tests do not diagnose lupus, then why are tests so important?

Tests, of and by themselves, do not make the diagnosis. They are helpful, though, as part of the diagnostic process, and they provide much important information to assist in developing treatment programs. Despite the fact that tests do not diagnose lupus, it is important to be aware of each of the tests that may be helpful as part of this process.

What are the eleven criteria for the diagnosis of lupus?

These eleven criteria for the classification of lupus were established in 1982 by a committee appointed by the American College of Rheumatology and were revised in 1998. They are as follows.

1. *Rash across the face.* A redness or rash on the face may appear in a butterfly configuration on the malar ridge or cheeks. It can appear on one or both sides of the face and is usually flat. Although there are times that this can be a discoid rash, it usually is not.

2. *Discoid rash.* This rash can involve blotches or raised scaly lesions. Scarring may result. These thick raised patches can occur on any part of the body.

3. *Sun sensitivity.* Lupus patients may experience a harmful physiological reaction to sunlight that is more severe than just a sunburn. The disease usually worsens with increased sun exposure in those who are sensitive.

4. *Ulcers in the mouth or nose.* Although mouth, nose, or throat ulcers or sores are not uncommon, frequent development of these sores may indicate lupus.

5. *Inflammation of joints.* Arthritic inflammation or pain in two or more joints can be a criterion of lupus. This inflammation is not accompanied by noticeable or marked deformity of these joints. Joint problems can show up as swelling, tenderness, or pain if the joint is moved. The joints that may be affected by these symptoms include those in the feet, ankles, fingers, knees, hips, elbows, shoulders, wrists, and jaw.

6. *Inflammation of the lining of the lungs or heart.* This is called *pleurisy* in the lungs and *pericarditis* in the heart. Pleurisy is the inflammation of the membrane that lines the inside of the chest cavity surrounding the lungs. Pericarditis is an inflammation of the sac or lining surrounding the heart.

7. *Kidney disorder.* There are two possible kidney problems that meet this criterion. The first is the existence of excessive protein in the urine (*proteinuria*). The other is the existence of cell *casts.* Casts are fragments of cells normally found in the blood, or fragments of the tubules of the kidney itself. If kidney disease exists, various casts may be found in the urine.

8. *Nervous system disorder.* Convulsions (seizures) or psychotic behavior can also be caused by drugs or a metabolic dysfunction. When this is not the case, this is a criterion for lupus.

9. *Blood system disorder.* This involves particular changes in the blood. These changes can include *hemolytic anemia,* wherein the red cells are coated with antibodies that cause them to break down and break apart; *leukopenia,* a low white blood count; *lymphopenia,* a decrease in the number of lymphocytes in the blood; or *thrombocytopenia,* low numbers of platelets in the blood.

10. *Immune disorder.* Two types of immune disorders that meet this criterion for lupus are the presence of the *LE cell* (a lupus ery-thematosus cell contains two nuclei rather than the one nucleus that cells usually have) and a false positive reaction to the test for syphilis. More recently, the presence of *antiphospholipid antibodies* has been added as an immune disorder than can be an indicator of lupus. Antiphospholipid antibodies are proteins directed against molecules called *phospholipids.* The phospholipids make up certain tissues and are part of a cell's membrane or covering.

11. *A positive ANA.* The body's production of *antinuclear antibodies* (antibodies that work against cell nuclei) is the final criterion for the diagnosis of lupus.

By consensus of experts, at least four of the eleven criteria should be present before a diagnosis of lupus is made.

Why is it necessary for a person to have at least four of the eleven criteria?

Although the criteria are often used to diagnose people with lupus, it was originally conceived as a tool for classifying patients for research. It is necessary that four of the eleven criteria be present in order to classify patients with lupus. The disease is so varied in its clinical presentation that four established criteria help to make sure that the patient actually has the disease.

COMMON TESTS FOR LUPUS

Is there one laboratory test that can diagnose all cases of lupus?

No. Lupus is a very complex illness. Cellular abnormalities abound, and these are difficult to detect. Moreover, their presence doesn't always guarantee that the patient has lupus. The antibody tests are generalized—in other words, they are not restricted to the lupus patient. Rather, they detect autoimmune phenomena that can be present in a variety of illnesses.

Are different tests available to diagnose which organ systems of the body are being affected by lupus?

Yes. Different tests, some immunologically based (based on cells or antibodies of the immune system) and some not, can help to determine which organs are affected. For example, lupus of the muscles can be diagnosed in three ways: detection of elevated released muscle enzymes (such as *creatine phosphokinase* or *aldolase*); the discovery of a specific antibody against the muscle fibers (such as *JO-1* or *Mi*); or physical tests like the *electromyogram* (*EMG*), a test of the electrical activity of muscles and nerves. Tests that are not necessarily associated with lupus (such as antithyroid, antiliver, and antiadrenal gland tests—tests that show antibodies being made against specific organ tissues) can also diagnose specific organ involvement. More often than not, immunologic tests cannot help one to distinguish this disease from other autoimmune diseases.

Tests commonly used in clinics can help to diagnose which organs are affected, but the ailments that these tests may detect may or may not be the result of lupus. These tests include blood sugar, blood urea nitrogen, and liver function tests.

What are the most commonly used tests in the diagnosis of lupus?

The *ANA, anti-DNA, anticardiolipin,* and *anti-Smith* (*Sm*) tests.

How often are these tests done?

Some of the tests (such as the anti-DNA, anticardiolipin, and the ANA) are done repeatedly. They are done with some frequency in a patient's life, due to the fact that the results of those tests may change over time. This helps the physician to better understand and monitor the disease.

The Smith, the RNP, the Ro, and the La antibody tests are not tests that are done repeatedly. They are usually done once or twice in the patient's history. They are used to ascertain whether or not these antibodies exist as part of the diagnosis. Once it is found that they do exist, it's not necessary to subsequently get more information on them.

The ANA (Antinuclear Antibodies) Test

What are antinuclear antibodies?

These are antibodies that, for some unknown reason, bind to the complex molecules that are present in the nucleus of each cell. There is no end to the array of proteins or other materials in the nucleus to which the antibody might be directed. There are literally thousands of molecules in the nucleus. We still do not understand why certain molecules are singled out as being "foreign" to the immune system.

How many different types of antinuclear antibodies are there?

There can be virtually thousands of different antinuclear antibodies. But there is a very specific amount of antinuclear antibody antigens in lupus—somewhere between eight and ten. The reason these antigens or materials in the nucleus become foreign to the immune system is unknown. Some of these antigens are DNA (both double-stranded and single-stranded); RNA; *Smith antigen* (a protein sugar named after a patient in whom it was first found, and found in 30 percent of patients with SLE); *ribonucleoprotein* (RNP); *histones* (small proteins around DNA on the chromosomes); *signal protein* (a protein involved in nucleus function in cells); and *Ro* and *La,* proteins in the nucleus. Some antibodies are also directed toward antigens in the *cytoplasm* (the cell sap that surrounds the nucleus or center of cell activity). These cytoplasmic antibodies are uncommon and are not grouped with the ANA.

What is the role of antinuclear antibodies in lupus?

There is none. It is believed that many specific antibodies (like the anti-DNA) form complexes that can cause damage to areas of the body like the *glomerulus* (the filtration apparatus of the kidney). These antibodies cause damage by causing destruction of filtration by making holes in the filter. Just why such immune complexes deposit in the kidney has been the subject of major investigation for many years. Immune complexes can—for no apparent reason—also deposit in places like the skin, with less severe effects. Immune complexes are composed of lots of antibody combined with antigen. The antigens are usually self-antigens like DNA, RNA, RNP, and so on, which are the targets of the antinuclear antibodies described earlier. Though most antinuclear antibodies are associated with lupus, they are not known to affect the disease process.

What is the connection between antinuclear antibodies and the LE cell?

The lupus (or LE) cell was described long before the antibody against nuclear material was discovered. Any cell coated with antibody is considered foreign by the immune system. These foreign substances are swallowed by a white cell and then deposited and destroyed in the spleen. Antinuclear antibody coats the nuclei of white cells and allows other white cells to believe that the coated cells are foreign and should be ingested. The *polymorphonuclear leukocyte* (PMN, a white cell that eats foreign materials or immune complexes) then swallows these coated white cells and becomes an LE cell. "Polymorphonuclear" means "many-formed nucleus." The LE cells are rarely sought in today's laboratories because they are not always found in lupus patients, and their absence does not necessarily mean that the patient does not have lupus. On the other hand, when discovered, they are very helpful in establishing a diagnosis.

What is the ANA test?

To measure a person's antinuclear antibodies, serum from the patient's blood is placed over a section of tissue derived from laboratory-grown cells, or taken from an animal. The antibody from the patient—if present—sticks to the nuclei of the cells in the tissue and causes them to fluoresce when treated with a special chemical. (This was once referred to as the *FANA,* or *fluorescent antinuclear antibody.*)

Is the ANA test the best currently available diagnostic test?

No. (There is no "best" diagnostic test!) The ANA is very inexpensive and easy to perform. However, it provides very general information. It merely gives one an overview of the patient's ability to make autoantibody. If the concentration (titer) of the ANA is determined to be very high, it is indicative of lupus or its closely related diseases. A positive ANA at low titer can often be found in normal people.

How reliable are tests for antinuclear antibodies?

This depends on the laboratory. The Committee for International Standardization of the ANA test meets often to deal with issues of reliability. Many variables can interfere with the ANA test and give false numbers and perhaps even a false diagnosis. The medium, or cells, used to measure the ANA is very important and varies from laboratory to laboratory. From the 1950s through the early 1980s, mouse or rat kidneys were used to look at these antibodies. Human liver tissue was also a reliable substrate (medium). Somewhere in the early 1980s, it became fashionable to use cultured laryngeal tumor cells (called Hep-2 cells) to measure the strength of the antibodies, and they are still used today.

Is this test always accurate?

No, for the reasons given earlier. The quality of the test depends on the substrate and other factors, including the strength of the fluorescent antibody and even the quality of the microscope being used.

What do the results of the ANA test determine?

Simply that the patient has antibody toward nuclear materials. The ANA can also be positive in "normal" people. For example, older individuals and pregnant women will have positive ANAs. People who take certain drugs (like procainamide and isoniazid) may also have positive ANAs without any signs or symptoms of any autoimmune disease, including lupus. Most patients with other diseases never achieve the high concentrations (titers) seen in the lupus patient. However, ANA titers in some patients with Sjogren's syndrome and overlap syndromes like mixed connective tissue disease have been reported to be very high.

How do the results of the ANA test determine what subsequent tests will be used?

We have what are called patterns of staining. The ANA test is always reported with a pattern as well as the strength. This pattern can be one of four kinds, or any combination of them. The four possible patterns are *diffuse* (the entire nucleus is stained); *speckled* (only a certain component of the nucleus is staining or acts as an antigen); *nucleolar* (usually indicates staining only of the nucleolus, or small nucleus within the larger nucleus); or *rim* (staining of the nuclear membrane, thought from the 1950s to the early 1980s to reflect DNA staining). Many experts feel that the only really helpful pattern is the nucleolar pattern, which often means that the patient has scleroderma (a disease where the skin and/or tissues in the body become thickened, usually due to a proliferation of collagen tissue).

Generally, the ANA should be positive before other antibodies (such as the anti-Smith or antiribonucleoprotein antibodies) are measured. Though the results of an ANA test is not the "end-all" of the lupus diagnosis, it can be helpful.

It used to be said that a negative ANA meant that lupus is not present. However, we now know that this is not the case. A patient can have both positive and negative ANA results during the course of the disease. If the ANA is positive, and the appropriate clinical signs are present, the patient should have further testing.

How many different types of antibodies are detected as part of ANA testing?

No one really knows. There are probably several antigens or materials in the nucleus that are targets for autoantibody (those proteins that are called antibodies that react with self tissues or molecules). There are billions of antigens in the body. Only a few of these react with antibodies. Far fewer react with autoantibodies. With further study, more autoantibodies will be discovered, as well as many yet undiscovered antigens to which lupus antibodies are directed.

How often do antinuclear antibodies appear?

It varies from patient to patient, even within the same family or between identical twins.

Why do the chances of a person testing positive on an ANA test increase with age?

No one really knows. It is generally believed that older people have decreased immune function, and it is this breakdown that allows for the formation of autoantibodies. Some call this *decreased immune surveillance.*

Is there such a thing as ANA-negative lupus?

No. Patients who do not have an antinuclear antibody may have been aggressively treated and lost the antibody titer or strength. The antibody must be positive over time in order for a patient to be classified as having lupus. Titers that are at a dilution of 1 to 80 or less are usually not considered positive.

Does the ANA just disappear?

Yes, the ANA can disappear over time when the patient is on drug therapy. The cell types that are used to show the antinuclear antibody's presence today are quite sensitive. It is therefore unusual to have lupus with a negative ANA, but it can happen. However, you should carry evidence of your positive test and certainly give a copy to your doctor.

The Anti-DNA Antibody Test

What is DNA and what role does it play in lupus?

DNA is the genetic material that is passed on from generation to generation. It exists in the cell nuclei of all individuals and is the matter that makes up genes. Patients with SLE can make antibodies to DNA. A person should not create antibody to DNA unless it is altered or coupled to some other substance, like a protein. This could happen via a chemical reaction. The fact that lupus patients create antibody to DNA in its unaltered form has puzzled scientists for years.

What is the anti-DNA antibody test?

This is the test that measures the amount of antibody made against DNA. DNA reacts with antibodies in people with lupus. If you inject DNA into animals without lupus, the animal receiving the injection cannot make antibody to this molecule. The immune system doesn't make antibody to materials that are *conserved* or fundamental in nature, and DNA is too fundamental a substance. In general, most people do not make antibody to DNA either, but people with lupus do.

In lupus patients, antibody to double-stranded DNA can be found. Single-strand DNA antibody also occurs, but this is not specific to lupus. So the antinative (double-stranded) DNA test helps us diagnose lupus. It is a fairly good predictor of the activity of the disease when organs like the kidneys are affected.

Generally, the DNA antibody detection test is done with radioactive DNA (so that any complexes that form will be radioactive and therefore easily detected and counted); with plain DNA and an enzyme test called ELISA (which causes a color change when antibodies bind to the DNA, making immune complexes easy to detect); or in a plate with many wells in which DNA is coated with sera. Care has to be taken to place only "native" or unbroken DNA in the wells, since the use of other DNA can result in a positive test. For some reason, many normal people have antibodies that stick to broken or single-stranded DNA. Because of this, the single-stranded DNA test is no longer used.

Do single-stranded DNA antibodies have any importance in SLE?

Single-stranded DNA antibodies are present in normal people and should never be followed as an index of clinical activity. The true antibody that reflects clinical activity is the antibody to native or double-stranded DNA.

The Anticardiolipin Antibody Test

What are anticardiolipin antibodies?

The *cardiolipin* molecule is an interesting phospholipid (a molecule that forms the basis of many tissues and membranes) associated with membranes in human cells, such as the inner *mitochondria* (mitochondria are structures within the cell that are responsible for the production of energy) and the membranes of certain bacteria.

There is a lack of cardiolipin in the rest of the body. For some strange reason, certain patients with lupus make antibodies to this molecule. Three kinds of anticardiolipin antibodies are possible: *IgG, IgM,* and *IgA*. Since it is currently easier to test for anticardiolipin antibodies than for the lupus anticoagulant (antibodies that are usually directed against platelets or certain clotting factors but in lupus actually *encourage* clotting to occur), this test is the one that is usually performed in small community hospitals. It is one of many antiphospholipid *assays* (laboratory tests or analyses in which antibodies to phospholipids are measured).

How is the anticardiolipin test performed?

It is performed by using the enzyme immunoassay (analysis). The phospholipids are placed in a dish, allowed to react with the patient's blood, and finally combined with a chemical that changes color. The intensity of color tells one how strong the reaction or concentration of antibody is in the patient.

The Anti-Smith (Sm) Test

What is the anti-Smith antibody?

The *anti-Smith antibody* is an antibody against a sugar protein. A patient named Smith was the first patient in whom this antibody was seen. (As is sometimes the case in medicine, antibodies are named after the patients in which they are first found.) The serum from the patient named Smith is still available and is used as a standard with which to compare other serums that have been derived over the years.

How often does the anti-Smith antibody appear?

The anti-Smith antibody is found in roughly 30 to 40 percent of patients with lupus. Some investigators believe that its presence can confirm the presence of lupus. This is contested, however, by others.

Under what circumstances would this test be performed?

This test would be performed when the diagnosis of lupus is initially suspected. It would be one of a series of tests being done. Remember, every piece of positive information that can be derived by doing any of these tests creates additional information that can lead the physician to a more accurate diagnosis of lupus.

How is the anti–Smith antibody test performed?

Anti–Smith antibody is measured in several ways. The antibody is in the sera of roughly 30 to 40 percent of lupus patients. It can be detected by taking the patient's blood and observing how it reacts with an isolated protein.

IMPORTANT FACTORS IN THE DIAGNOSIS OF LUPUS

The following other factors, components, tests, and diagnostic procedures are also important to understand.

The LE Factor

What is the LE factor and the LE phenomenon?

The *LE factor* refers to the actual autoantibody that causes one cell to "eat" another. The LE factor is the antibody, and the *LE phenomenon* is the process of one cell eating another (*autophagocytosis*).

What is the LE cell prep test?

The LE cell test used to be performed with some regularity. It involved mixing the white cells of a lupus patient with the white cells of someone without the disease. The normal white cells would ingest the cell nuclei of the patient who did not have lupus. The test was performed using the cells of a patient *suspected* of having lupus. When the cells of the person known not to have lupus ingested the others, the result was considered to be positive.

The LE test is a very difficult test to perform. It used to be employed before we knew anything about fluorescent antibody techniques. However, the LE test produces a lot of false negatives (patients who had auto-antibodies were often found not to have LE cells in their blood). On the other hand, there were very few false positives. So when the test was positive it was really helpful.

This test is infrequently done today because of its complexity, because of the fact that technicians have to be specifically trained to do it, and because it is somewhat difficult to perform since you need normal white cells (which don't live very long) from other people.

Complement

What is complement?

Complement is the name for a series of proteins found in the blood that amplifies immune reactions. There are nine such proteins (C1–C9). Each of these proteins may have subgroups. For example, complement component 1 has at least three parts: C1s, C1r, and C1q. The letters are assigned just to differentiate the components of complement. Occasionally, and for unknown reasons, some people have genetic deficiencies of the complement components. A large percentage (approximately 90 percent) of these people eventually acquire autoimmune diseases. Lupus is the most common of these.

For example, those patients with C1q deficiency are prone to acquiring a lupus-like syndrome that can be quite deadly. Its symptoms include skin lesions and a form of chronic obstructive pulmonary disease. Patients can inherit the deficiency in either a *homozygous* (genes for C1q are missing from each chromosome) or a *heterozygous* (only one gene for C1q is missing) manner. Those with a heterozygous deficiency are less affected. Other hereditary deficiencies include C2, C3, and C4. Deficiencies of C5 through C9 are not associated with lupus-like illness. They are usually linked to an increased risk of certain infections.

When a person experiences an immune system reaction, this reaction consumes complement components. That's why complement components are low when measured in people with active lupus.

What, then, is the role of complement in diagnosing lupus?

Measurement of complement is routinely used to see whether a person has a component deficiency. Because this may be a problem for someone with lupus, this deficiency can play a role in the cumulative information used in diagnosing and monitoring lupus.

When a complement level is low because the complement is used up in an immune complex that forms, the person can be quite ill. The levels of complement can be normalized with treatment and form a basis with which to measure the effectiveness of treatment. Complement component deficiency due to lupus activity has to be compared to the rare complement deficiency on the basis of heredity. Complement deficiency, when it is genetic, is often associated with the onset of lupus-like illness in early adulthood. Remember that most of the complement loss seen in the lupus patient is the result of consumption, or use, of the complement in an immune reaction.

What diagnostic procedure is used for complement?

The CH50 is a very useful blood test. This test measures the overall function of complement. It actually determines whether a patient has any complement available to *lyse* (explode or destroy) guinea pig or sheep cells coated with antibody. Such cells are used in the test because they are foreign to the human immune system.

If the cells explode in the test tube, it means that the patient's complement is functioning normally. If the sheep cells or guinea pig cells don't explode, the patient does not have normal levels of complement. This means that the complement is being bound up by immune complexes caused by lupus, is being removed from circulation, and therefore is not available to explode the cells in the test tube. Anybody with lupus who has a superlow complement has very active disease. The exception would be someone with hereditary component deficiency.

What is the difference between low complement and complement deficiency, and why is this important?

Complement deficiency is usually due to a genetic flaw that results in nonproduction of complement. This is different from the low complement that results from lupus activity binding complement to immune complexes. It is often difficult for physicians to distinguish between these two reasons for low complement level. This is important because a doctor might erroneously treat a patient with strong drugs for some time, waiting for the complement level to rise, when in fact it is not possible to raise.

What is the significance of C3 and C4 in the test of serum complements?

The C3 and C4 are specific components of complement that are measured. The test helps the clinician determine what mechanism may or may not be involved in the development of lupus by determining which of the specific components is missing. In other words, which of the two components is missing has different implications for the clinician who is trying to determine what is going on. For example, a missing C3 component may occur in individuals who have severe lupus involving the kidneys, the brain, or the skin (usually because the C3 component is attached to immune complexes that are most widely consumed in the brain, kidney, or skin).

What does it mean if my C4 is low and my C3 is normal?

The C4 component of complement is a part of the alternate system. The location of the C4 gene on chromosome 6 means that it has some special importance, as most of the immune response genes are on chromosome 6. However, only two components of complement come from genes on that chromosome, C2 and C4. There is such a thing as a patient with C4 that is not up to normal levels, called a *C4 null patient*, who is predisposed to autoimmune disease. More important, if the C4 and C3 are both depleted due to consumption by immune complexes, it may indicate active disease.

Are there complement deficiencies that mean that I will get lupus?

There are several complement deficiencies that are associated with the onset of lupus, including C2 deficiency and C1q deficiency. These deficiencies are very rare, but they must be mentioned because they are often missed by physicians. Other components of complement can be depleted, and this depletion is associated with some lupus-like autoimmune diseases.

What are the best tests that my doctor can order routinely at one sitting?

The tests that mean something to the lupus patient and those that most physicians order for quick results are the antinative DNA antibody assay and the total hemolytic complement. The total hemolytic complement is known as the CH 50 or the CH 100.

Sed Rate

What is the sedimentation (or sed) rate?

The *sed rate* or *ESR* is an abbreviation for the *erythrocyte sedimentation rate.* The test for this measures the level of *plasma fibrinogen,* a protein that makes the red blood cells clump together. It is elevated when a patient is ill and/or has some type of general inflammation.

What role does it play in lupus?

The sed rate is usually elevated in lupus patients, though an elevated sed rate is not specific to lupus patients.

What diagnostic procedures are used to test the sed rate?

The test for the sedimentation rate is really quite simple. Blood is drawn, placed into a very small tube called a capillary tube, and spun in a modified *centrifuge* (a device used to separate substances in a liquid). The red cells fall into a pile, either slowly or quickly. When the red cells settle toward the bottom of the tube, they leave a large area of clear plasma. This area is measured over one hour.

The more plasma that is left, the greater the sedimentation rate. The normal range is usually less than 30 millimeters per hour. An elevated sed rate means that there is a lot of inflammatory activity going on in the body. Measurement can assist in the diagnosis and detection of inflammatory conditions. It is also a good way to follow lupus activity.

Can the sedimentation rate be normal when I am very sick?

In rare instances the sedimentation rate can be normal when someone is sick. The sedimentation rate represents plasma fibrinogen made by the liver. If one has liver disease, one may not have a significantly elevated sedimentation rate.

Rheumatoid Factor

What is the rheumatoid factor?

An autoantibody that is more commonly found in rheumatoid arthritis, the *rheumatoid factor* (*RF*) rarely occurs in someone with lupus. In fact, when it occurs in a patient with lupus it is very interesting because lupus patients should not have rheumatoid factors. We've mentioned this simply because many people with lupus have heard about the rheumatoid factor and have asked questions about what it means to them. The answer? Very little.

Can the rheumatoid factor be useful to the lupus patient if it is positive?

Although the rheumatoid factor test is not specific for lupus and does not correlate with clinical activity for lupus, it is routinely done for many lupus patients. A positive rheumatoid factor assay is rarely seen in lupus but is commonly found in related autoimmune diseases such as rheumatoid arthritis and Sjogren's syndrome.

VISUALIZATION PROCEDURES

There are a number of visualization techniques that are helpful to doctors in the diagnosis of lupus. Generally, doctors like to progress from the simplest to the more technically advanced procedures. An explanation follows of each of these procedures.

What is the progression of visualization procedures used, and what do they involve?

The progression of complexity and cost usually moves from ultrasound, to X-ray, to CAT scan, to MRI. Which procedure is used depends on the degree of accuracy necessary.

Ultrasound

Visualization starts with *ultrasound,* the technique that produces the sonogram, and involves bouncing sound waves off the organ. It's noninvasive, and it's very inexpensive. This procedure, also called *sonography,* can be very useful. The ultrasound machine, which often resembles a microphone, is brought into the examining room. Jelly is put on the patient in the area that is going to be examined, and the microphone is moved back and forth, emitting sound waves that are reflected into the machine. When the microphone is in the appropriate position, the reflected sound waves form a picture of the organ on a computer-like screen. The doctor then makes some still photographs of the result using a Polaroid.

X-rays

If the ultrasound doesn't give us the required information or is not appropriate for the area being examined, we might look at *X-rays.* In an X-ray, the patient is placed next to a photographic plate. When the X-ray is taken, a picture is made on the plate and the plate gets developed into what we know as the X-ray film.

CAT Scans

A *CAT* (*computerized axial tomogram*) is focused X-ray technology that is used to help define structures within the body when an X-ray doesn't reveal enough information. The CAT scan is also used to do procedures such as a biopsy with accuracy. For a conventional CAT scan, a patient lies on the table as X-rays are shot around the periphery of an organ or part of the body. Instead of the X-ray being developed as a film, the pictures appear as computerized images on the computer screen.

A spiral CAT scan is a special form of CAT scan that involves the continuous movement of patients through a scanner that produces a higher definition of internal structures. The spiral CAT scan permits greater visualization of blood vessels and internal tissues and is particularly useful for imaging the chest cavity.

Contrast is often added to the CAT scan in order to increase sensitivity or help make a diagnosis. In some instances the addition of contrast might be harmful to the patient, as when a patient is dehydrated or allergic to the dye. Your doctor knows when this is the case.

MRI

Magnetic resonance imagery (*MRI*) is the ultimate process used in diagnostic detection and visualization of organs and tissues.

What does a person experience during an MRI?

MRIs are usually done in special rooms in special chambers. In an MRI (like with a CAT scan), you lie on a table, but this one slides inside a chamber. Then a (relatively noisy) machine bounces X-rays off the atoms and molecules in your body, and a computer takes the atomic vibrations and reassembles them on a screen so that we're actually looking at your organ, such as the kidneys, liver, pancreas, or spleen. You don't feel anything; you only hear the noise. The MRI pictures can give information about not only the structure of the tissue but also its density. They can also tell whether a mass is liquid or solid.

Some patients don't like the claustrophobia-like feeling of being in a chamber. But because the magnetic resonance is very sensitive, the patient has to be in a very special, closed (confined) chamber in order to have the MRI work. In most cases, the doctors and technicians involved in the MRI process will do everything they can to help you to be more comfortable during the procedure. There are such things as "open" MRIs, where the chamber is more open and less confining, but there have been cases in which the definition of the computer-generated pictures is not as good as those produced in the closed MRI.

Metal objects such as metal teeth and plates in the head or bones cannot be placed in an MRI machine. Vibrations from a train or a truck going by on a highway will ruin the clarity of an MRI.

Exactly how does the MRI work?

This process utilizes a high-intensity visualization machine that involves the complex principle of atomic vibration. When all the atoms in a tissue or organ of the body are vibrating in a field at different intensity levels, they create different patterns on a computer screen. This can determine the density of objects.

Why is the MRI so helpful?

By using the MRI, we can see things today that we could never see in the past, in an almost three-dimensional way. It provides a tremendous opportunity to look at pathology without cutting the person open.

What role does the MRI play in diagnosing lupus?

The MRI is not routinely used to diagnose lupus. However, the MRI is helpful in a number of instances. It may be used in the head to look at the brain to see if there are tumors, hemorrhages, or clots in the brain, or to see if there is inflammation in the brain. It may be used when it is necessary to study joint spaces (if tendons and/or other fine structures must be looked at) to see if there is fluid in the joints. It's particularly useful in lupus patients when doctors are looking for avascular necrosis, or the death of the heads or the body of bones as a result of the anti-phospholipid antibodies or steroid therapy. There are other instances where the MRI may be used as well, such as in the abdomen to look at the liver, gallbladder, pancreas, spleen, adrenal glands, and kidneys. It's usually up to the doctor whether or not to use MRI, and it depends on the symptoms reported.

MRI is usually the last visualization procedure to be used. Only in very special, medically determined circumstances is the MRI used earlier in the "hierarchy." If there are problems in the head, CAT scans and MRIs may be used sooner, because skull X-rays do not visualize the brain, and ultrasound is useless in the head.

What is an MRA?

A *magnetic resonance angiogram* (*MRA*) reveals the vessels of the brain by imaging the overall flow of blood in the brain. It does not involve needles or the injection of dyes and it is fast. An MRA is performed when one or a series of small strokes is suspected to have occurred.

BIOPSIES

What is a biopsy?

A *biopsy* is the removal of a tiny piece of the patient's tissue so that it can be sent for microscopic examination.

What types of biopsies are done on lupus patients and why?

Biopsies can serve many purposes in the diagnosis of lupus. The first useful biopsy is the renal or kidney biopsy. This is useful in predicting the course of certain renal lesions, localizing the kind of antibody deposition in the kidney's filtration mechanism, and judging the degrees of *chronicity* (how long a lesion has been present) and *activity* (how treatable a certain lesion is) of a person's kidney lupus. A biopsy of the kidney is recommended prior to instituting hard-core chemotherapy (more about this in chapter 5). The biopsy is usually performed with a fine needle. In certain instances, it must be performed in an operating room under anesthesia because of the risk of bleeding or other possible complications.

A second major biopsy for lupus patients is the skin biopsy. This is called the *band test*. The skin is tested to see if antibodies, immunoglobulins, and/or complement components are deposited in the skin. If the band test is positive, it usually means that the patient has lupus.

A third kind of useful biopsy is the muscle biopsy. This is often combined with the skin biopsy. It can often tell the reasons for muscle weakness and its primarily done in two circumstances: either when an EMG is positive (meaning that the patient has either nerve or muscle disease), or if the patient has muscle enzymes in the blood (the result of muscle fiber lysis—or destruction—due to an immune attack).

SOME COMMON CONCERNS

What is the role of a complete blood count as a diagnostic procedure?

A complete blood count should be performed regularly in the lupus patient. This is because a decrease of white cells (leukocytes, lymphocytes, or other cells) can signal trouble. Antibodies against these cells can reduce their numbers. Moreover, a rise in the white count can mean infection, and is, therefore, helpful in differentiating lupus from infection. However, the most important part of a blood count is the measurement of the platelet count. Platelets are important to the clotting of blood. Low platelet counts, which are often a problem in lupus, need to be carefully monitored.

Why look at the platelets?

The *platelets* are particles that are involved in the clotting process. They are not cells but rather fragments of cells. They come from a larger cell that is produced in the bone marrow. If you have low platelets, it means that you have a propensity to bleed. Platelet depletion in lupus rarely gets to levels where it is a danger to the patient. However, if the platelet level drops below 20,000, a patient may have to be treated in order to raise the platelet level. The platelets are often removed by antiplatelet antibodies, and drugs that cause immunosuppression may have to be added to raise the platelet levels.

What tests are used to detect immune complexes in the blood?

There are both very expensive and inexpensive tests to find immune complexes in blood. Tests like the *C1q,* testing for the level of this specific complement component; the *Raji,* testing using cells that have complement and Fc receptors (the Fc component is the tail of the heavy chain of an antibody molecule that sticks to other antibodies) on their surfaces; or a variety of other immune system assays or analyses can determine the presence of complexes. However, there is not much clinical usefulness for these tests, because any autoantibody test that is positive suggests that immune complexes are present in a patient's blood.

What is the role of urinalysis?

Urinalysis, the laboratory analysis of urine, is helpful in determining whether there are kidney abnormalities or pathology. For example, certain cells can be found, by themselves or in clumps called casts, in the urine of some patients. These casts indicate kidney disease. The level of the kidney disease can be determined from this and other tests.

What is a blood protein analysis?

There are two kinds. One measures the *serum albumin,* a substance found in large concentration in the blood that is necessary to control blood volume. This test gives an indication of the extent and duration of disease. A low albumin usually suggests a chronic disease. The second test measures the *gamma globulin* (the immunizing fraction of the blood protein) levels by testing the level of a patient's proteins. A high total protein in a lupus patient usually means that the patient has a high gamma globulin level, which means that the patient's immune system is very active. Patients with lupus usually have a very high gamma globulin level. Rarely is a patient with lupus *hypogammaglobulinemic* (having a low gamma globulin level). Hypogammaglobulinemic patients have immunodeficiencies—their immune systems are not active enough.

Why do some people with lupus have a false-positive test for syphilis?

It is not exactly known. It is believed, however, that it is because the syphilis organism is partially made up of phospholipids. The phospholipids that are found in lupus are the same compounds that would give a positive test for syphilis. It doesn't mean that the patient has ever had syphilis. It means that the antibody in the serum can't tell the difference. It is actually the patient's antiphospholipid antibody that's reacting with the material in the syphilis test.

What is the importance of antiphospholipid antibodies?

Frequent miscarriages and early fetal loss have been associated with the presence of antiphospholipid antibodies. Patients with frequent abortions are considered high-risk patients and should probably be tested for both anticardiolipin antibody and lupus anticoagulant. A marker for these antibodies is an elevated *PTT* (*partial thromboplastin time*). This is a test that measures clotting time. A patient can have antiphospholipid antibodies without having actual lupus erythematosus. This is called *primary antiphospholipid syndrome* and is more common in men.

What are immunoglobulins?

Immunoglobulins are protein molecules acting as antibodies that belong to a certain family of proteins. (In fact, the two terms, *immunoglobulins* and *antibodies,* can be used interchangeably.) Occasionally, they react with self antigens, as in those found in the lupus patient or patients with other autoimmune diseases. There are millions of antibodies that circulate in the serum, and they are the policemen of the immune system. When someone is reexposed to a foreign substance many years after initial exposure, the immune system has a memory that announces the return of the foreign material. A specific antibody is called up by the immune system in vast amounts to deal with the challenge of the antigen again.

What is the lupus anticoagulant?

The *lupus anticoagulant* is a very confusing antibody that was once thought to make patients bleed. That is why it was called an anticoagulant. There are, indeed, antibodies in lupus patients that can result in bleeding, but they are not the lupus anticoagulants. These "bleeding" antibodies are usually directed against platelets or certain clotting factors. Conversely, the lupus anticoagulant is a molecule that actually encourages clotting to occur. This makes it, in fact, a procoagulant, rather than an anticoagulant; but the name remains.

What are the PT and PTT, and what are their significance?

The *PT* is the *prothrombin time.* This is the measure of one pathway of clotting or coagulation of blood. It is the most useful test to measure the effect of the blood thinners Coumadin or warfarin. An elevated PT could mean many things. In a lupus patient on an anticoagulant it is useful to measure the clotting time. In the absence of anticoagulants, an elevated PT might mean that there is significant liver disease.

The PTT is the partial thromboplastin time. It measures a different clotting pathway than the PT. The PTT is often used to measure the effects of heparin on clotting. It is also abnormally high when a patient has a lupus anticoagulant. An elevated PTT can be more significant than elevated PT in lupus. The most important aspect of the PTT is its elevation when there is a lupus anticoagulant. This is often the first sign of the antiphospholipid syndrome.

Are there any differences in the diagnosis of lupus in children?

No. The diagnostic tests are the same—the patients are just smaller!

3.

Symptoms of Lupus

· ·

There are many symptoms of lupus. Some people have some of them, but no one has all of them. Most only have a few. But regardless of the symptoms you have, you probably have questions about what they are and how they can affect you. This chapter will attempt to answer these questions, providing you with valuable information about the variety of symptoms that occur in lupus.

What are the most common symptoms of lupus?

Although in lupus virtually any medical symptom can arise and the cause be mistaken for something else, there are certain specific symptoms that should alert one that the cause may be lupus. These include prolonged low-grade fever, joint pain or inflammation, weakness and fatigue, sudden loss of hair, and ulcers in the nose and mouth. Other symptoms that have been associated with the disease are as follows: weight loss; anemia; sun-sensitive rash; *Raynaud's phenomenon* (the toes and the fingers turn red, white, and blue because spasms in their small arteries stop the blood flow); inflammation of the membranes around the lungs, heart, or abdomen; seizures; phlebitis (inflammation of the wall of a vein); recurrent miscarriages during pregnancy; psychosis (a pathological mental disorder marked by loss of contact with reality); and kidney inflammation.

What are the categories of lupus symptoms?

Symptoms of lupus can be divided into several categories. No one ever has all the symptoms. Most people have only a few symptoms.

- *General symptoms.* Weakness, fatigue, low-grade fevers, generalized aching, and chills are included in this category.
- *Skin.* Skin problems include rashes, patchy lesions, and red inflammations. Scarring on the scalp may cause hair loss.
- *Chest.* Symptoms involving the chest include chest pain due to pleurisy or pericarditis. Both of these conditions may cause difficulty breathing, pain, shortness of breath, and a rapid heartbeat. Inflammation in the rib area or in the abdominal muscles may cause chest pain as well.
- *Muscular system.* Symptoms include weakness, aches, and pain.
- *Joints.* Joint symptoms include arthritis-like pain, swelling, redness, and stiffness.
- *Blood.* Blood symptoms include a low red blood cell count (anemia), decreased white blood cell counts (leading to increased susceptibility to infection), increased amounts of gamma globulin, and a false positive test for syphilis.
- *Cardiac or circulatory system.* Symptoms include increased swelling of the extremities, accumulation of fluid in the sac surrounding the heart, and Raynaud's phenomenon.
- *Digestive system.* Symptoms include stomach pain, cramps, nausea, vomiting, diarrhea, and constipation.
- *Kidneys.* Decreased kidney filtering efficiency leads to *uremia* (increased waste products remaining in circulation). Another symptom is proteinuria (excessive amounts of protein lost in the urine).
- *Nervous system.* Various parts of the nervous system, including the brain, spinal cord, and nerves, may be involved. Symptoms include headaches, or in more severe cases, seizures, temporary paralysis, psychotic behavior, or stroke.

Which are the earliest symptoms of lupus for physicians to detect?

The earliest symptoms are often flu-like ones. The patient will experience fatigue and exhaustion accompanied by sporadic joint discomfort. There may also be a rash. The rash, which can itch or burn, is associated with recent sun exposure and is usually located on the face or arms.

Which symptoms appear later and are more difficult to detect?

Physicians generally have no clues to the presence of kidney or brain disease caused by lupus until the organs are severely affected. When lupus affects the heart and lungs, the disease can cause mild shortness of breath or heart irregularity without the patient or physician knowing the actual cause.

Are any symptoms more common in children than in adults, or vice versa?

No. There are no symptoms that appear to be common to a specific age group.

Why do symptoms vary from person to person?

No one knows why symptoms vary from person to person. It's probably because every person is different, so everyone is affected by the disease in a different way.

Q Why do symptoms vary within the same person? Why may a person have one symptom, or group of symptoms, at one time in the course of lupus and other symptoms at different times?

Again, no one knows.

Q If one's symptoms are in one specific area (for example, musculoskeletal), are those the only symptoms that that person will experience?

The answer is no. The disease can manifest itself in any number of ways and at any particular time. Although it is not likely that more than one major organ system will be affected, there have been many patients with multiorgan involvement. For example, a patient might have joint, skin, and kidney involvement. It is hoped that if there is multiorgan involvement, this does not include vital organs that are indispensable for life.

Q Is it true that any symptoms experienced in the first two years are more than likely the only ones that will ever be experienced?

No, unfortunately that is not true. Although normally symptoms remain in the same systems, one must be constantly vigilant for new signs and symptoms. This is because the type of antibodies produced and the organs of the body that are affected by autoimmune reactions can change.

COMPLICATIONS OF THE JOINTS AND MUSCLES

How can lupus affect the joints?

Lupus generally causes some degree of joint pain without causing erosion of the bones. Lupus causes inflammation of the lining of the joint. Inflammatory chemicals are secreted by the cells in the joint (they are provoked by the body's inflammatory response to immune complexes), so that the joint gets red hot and swollen. The same thing occurs in other joint diseases. The difference is that in lupus, although there is destruction of soft tissue around the joints (like tendons), the bones are not destroyed. Patients with rheumatoid arthritis have significant joint inflammation but have bone erosions as well. Less than 5 percent of lupus patients have bony erosions. (This 5 percent is said to have "rhupus"—a hybrid disease of lupus and rheumatoid arthritis!)

How common are arthritic symptoms in lupus?

Over 90 percent of patients with lupus will, at some point, experience arthritic symptoms.

How do doctors determine whether or not joint problems are associated with lupus?

Doctors examine various parts of the joints during an exam. They first look for swelling, redness, and the appearance of fluid. They also check for symmetry—whether or not the opposite joint is affected in the patient. It's also important to count the number of joints that are affected to make sure the patient has lupus rather than another related rheumatologic disease. SLE involves most joints, and they can be inflamed like rheumatoid arthritic joints, but they are often nonsymmetrically affected. If a doctor can remove fluid from the inflamed joint, the number of cells and the character of the fluid can often tell the doctor the nature of the disease. Other aids like X-rays can help by detecting bone erosions, since erosions are rarely found in SLE joints. Range of motion is also a factor that is measured.

What joints are usually affected?

All joints can be affected. However, lupus most commonly affects the fingers, wrists, elbows, shoulders, knees, and feet. The spine and hips are usually not affected in the early stages. When hip pain does occur, it is usually due to a condition called *aseptic necrosis* (death of tissue without infection). This can be either a complication of the disease or an effect of drug therapy with steroids.

What exactly causes joint pain?

Where there is an immune reaction to the joint, the presence of immune complexes (the autoantibody and autoantigen combinations) attracts white cells to the area. (This is a process called *chemoattraction*.) These white cells have receptors on their surfaces that trigger mechanisms that cause the release of inflammatory chemicals (mediators). Joint pain is caused by the inflammatory chemicals released by white cells.

What causes the swelling of joints?

As mentioned earlier, inflammatory chemicals are released by white cells and cause joint pain. In addition, they also trigger a fluid leakage from the blood vessels into the joint fluid. This buildup of fluid is what we know as the swelling of the affected joint and can also contribute to the pain.

What is synovitis?

The joint is lined with cells called *synoviocytes*. The lining itself is referred to as the *synovial lining*. When this lining becomes inflamed, it is called *synovitis*.

Is damage to the joints reversible?

It is, to a degree. Only soft tissues are affected by the inflammation. This causes little joint destruction or erosion of bone. However, destruction of tendons or joint coverings can occur, and this can lead to significant deformity of the joint. Many patients develop deformities and require braces or other apparatus for stability and alignment. However, this kind of joint deformity does not occur in the vast majority of patients, for unknown reasons.

Is lupus a type of arthritis?

No. However, arthritis can be a symptom of lupus.

What is the difference between the arthritis in lupus and osteoarthritis or rheumatoid arthritis?

In *osteoarthritis* (also called degenerative arthritis), there is bone growth and destruction of cartilage. In rheumatoid arthritis, there is bone erosion with significant irreversible deformity. In lupus, "leaching of bone" (known as *osteoporosis*—calcium loss in the bone) and soft tissue inflammation can occur, but destruction of the actual joint is not very common.

How are joint problems treated in lupus?

Joint problems are most often treated with anti-inflammatory drugs called NSAIDs (nonsteroidal anti-inflammatory drugs).

Are steroids used for arthritic symptoms?

Generally, no. However, some physicians do use steroids for arthritis when it is particularly severe or painful and there is the threat of significant deformity.

How can lupus affect the muscles?

Antibodies and white cells may be directed against muscle cells, resulting in lysis, or complete destruction of the muscle. The cells that can attack muscle cells are called *cytotoxic lymphocytes* (or those that will kill other cells). Sometimes, actual antibodies attached to certain parts of the muscle can be observed in a test called immunofluorescence of muscle. This test is generally performed by taking blood from a patient and causing it to react with the muscle of another person or an animal to see whether there is antibody in the blood directed against muscle. What we want to do is find out if the muscle cells have antibodies attached to them. This would indicate that there are autoantibodies to muscle.

How often do muscle problems occur in lupus?

It is generally believed that the muscles of almost all people with active lupus are affected in some manner. However, in some individuals, *myositis* (inflammation of the muscle) is a chief symptom of the disease.

What happens when muscles become inflamed due to lupus?

Generally, the muscles located near the center of the body—the muscles in the upper arms and the thighs—(called the proximal, or near, muscles of the body) are the first to be affected. They first burn and become quite painful, and then they become very weak.

How do doctors test for muscle problems?

There are several steps in testing. The first is the clinical exam. Clinical testing determines if the muscles are weak and if the nerves are functioning properly. This is done through tests of reflexes, vibration sense, and sensation. Next, a blood test is performed that examines the levels of creatine phosphokinase (CPK) and aldolase in the blood. Measuring the levels of these enzymes shows just how much muscle injury is present. Last, an EMG (electromyogram) electrically measures the amount of muscle damage by measuring electrical impulses from the muscles.

How can lupus flares lead to loss of muscle tone?

Loss of muscle tone can occur for two reasons: the actual inflammation or the overall effects of steroid hormones on muscle function (*steroid myopathy*).

Why is this important to treat?

It is important to treat lupus myositis to prevent the complete destruction of muscles that would cause loss of tone and strength. In steroid myopathy, the muscles can become infiltrated with fat, and the patient can develop significant weakness and loss of strength.

How are muscle problems treated?

Muscle problems are treated differently, depending on the stage of the disease. First, steroid hormones are administered to reverse destruction of the muscles. It then becomes very important to build the muscle tone with regular physical therapy or exercise. The therapy and exercise should be done under the supervision of a physician.

Aches and Pains

Why does lupus cause achiness?

This is usually the result of inflammation of muscles or joints.

How long do aches and pains usually last?

They may persist until the patient is sufficiently treated and the immune response or disease process that is causing the pain is weakened or removed. If not treated, they could last forever.

What can be done to ease the pain?

Most patients who have lupus with aches and pains take pain relievers like Tylenol (acetaminophen). They can take low doses of aspirin, over-the-counter antiinflammatories, or even prescription pain medicines like Darvon (propoxyphene hydrochloride). Most of these medications help the aches and pains of lupus. In addition to medication, other activities such as physical therapy, exercise, or even psychological techniques can be used to ease pain (see chapters 4 and 5).

Why does lupus create tenderness?

Tenderness is a result of inflammation and of the migration of white cells that release the inflammatory chemicals that can cause tissue destruction to the site of injury or immune reaction. These white cells secrete chemicals that cause more white cells to migrate out of the blood vessels and into the joint. Consequently, large amounts of inflammatory materials (such as histamine, serotonin, and slow reactive substances) accumulate in the joint. These materials can be made in the laboratory. If injected into the skin, the skin would become red, swollen, and painful. Similar processes occur in the joints.

What are arthralgia and myalgia?

Arthralgia is joint pain, and *myalgia* is muscle pain.

What is fibromyalgia?

Fibromyalgia is a painful, debilitating disease affecting the muscles that usually occurs by itself. Nobody really knows what causes it. Many scientists believe that it is a disorder of the pain proteins in nerves and muscles. Some people think it's a muscle disorder. Some think it's an innate nerve disorder with abnormal secretion of certain proteins. Some believe that it is related to thyroid function in a way that is as yet unknown or to lack of adrenal function. Some think that the disease is purely psychological in nature. The psychological hypothesis seems unlikely since the disease is very predictable in patients who have certain symptom patterns; namely trigger points (areas of the skin or muscle that experience pain when pressure is applied) that are found in specific locations throughout the body. It would be very difficult (although not totally impossible) to reproduce these symptoms psychologically. Moreover, the symptoms can be relieved with topical anesthetics in most instances, which would probably not be the case if the condition was psychological. All we really know is that fibromyalgia causes a pain pattern, a sleep disorder, and sometimes, a personality disturbance.

What is the treatment for fibromyalgia in SLE?

Fibromyalgia can be treated with many different kinds of drugs, but it never responds to nonsteroidal anti-inflammatory drugs (NSAIDs) or corticosteroids. The treatment of fibromyalgia includes anaerobic exercise, tricyclic antidepressants to allow the patient to sleep, and analgesic agents to relieve pain.

What is the danger of having fibromyalgia pain with lupus?

For unknown reasons fibromyalgia and SLE often occur together. The danger of having both conditions at the same time is that your doctor may mistake the fibromyalgia pain for lupus joint or muscle pain and increase your steroids like prednisone or cortisone. Since patients with fibromyalgia do not usually respond to steroids, the patient can be on very high doses of steroids for no reason as the fibromyalgia pain persists.

Why are you discussing fibromyalgia in a book about lupus?

The reason we're discussing fibromyalgia in this book is that it can also occur in patients with lupus. It is not a symptom of lupus; it is a separate disease that can also occur (with some frequency) in people with lupus.

The cause of this disorder in lupus patients is not clear. Many patients who have fibromyalgia with lupus experience insomnia and increased sensitivity to light. Fortunately, fibromyalgia is not life-threatening, but it is very distressing to the patient.

What is the role of exercise in the treatment of muscle or joint pain in lupus?

It is very important to keep muscles and joints active for a variety of reasons. First, muscles must be toned in order to function adequately. The size of the muscle and its blood circulation depend on where the muscle is and what it does. The main reason for isometric aerobic exercise (oxygen-consuming exercise) is to increase the tone and bulk of muscles. Patients with fibromyalgia may have to be careful with regard to isometric exercise. While oxygen in the muscle is increased, the pain of doing such an exercise might preclude any derived benefit. Aerobic exercises like walking or swimming are much better for all patients with lupus and any accompanying fibromyalgia. Physical therapy performed with the aid of an expert therapist may be very beneficial to the patient who is trying to maintain muscle integrity and tone. Joints depend on tendons and the calcification of the bones. These, in turn, depend on continued movement. Significant bone loss through osteoporosis occurs when the bones are not used regularly. People who require long periods of bed rest are at risk for osteoporosis.

SKIN COMPLICATIONS

What are the skin symptoms of lupus?

The skin symptoms are so varied that lupus's expression in the skin is one of the most mysterious aspects of the disease. Symptoms can range from a simple, painful rash to itchy hives to deep ulcerations that can significantly disfigure the patient. Whether or not these disfigurements are permanent depends on the location and severity of the lesion.

What is a lesion?

A *lesion* is a change in tissue due to injury or disease.

What is a rash?

A *rash* is inflammation of the skin.

What exactly causes rashes in lupus?

No one really knows. Biopsies of the skin of lupus patients show immune complexes at the junction or connection of the *dermal-epidermal membrane,* a significant site in the skin for growth and regeneration, which could be perceived as a cause. However, all patients with lupus have immune complexes in their skin, yet only a small percentage of those with lupus have rashes due to sun sensitivity (approximately 35 to 50 percent or more). Hence the cause of rashes is still unknown.

How many different types of skin problems are there?

Lupus can have numerous effects on the skin. However, none of these effects alone necessarily mean that you have lupus.

The effects include:

- Discoid lesions (flat, mildly ulcerated, nonpainful, scaly lesions that occur on sun-exposed areas)
- Blush rashes (warm and mildly tender rashes that look like a blush or a vasodilated area)
- Malar facial rashes (rashes on the face above the cheeks)
- Blood vessel lesions (spider-like marks on the skin, inflammation of the small blood vessels, blood clots under the skin causing swelling, constrictive lesions like those seen in Raynaud's phenomenon, chronic ulceration, nodules, and sometimes gangrene)
- Hair loss (both generalized and patchy)
- Lesions in the mouth, nose, or vagina
- Itchy hives (raised and itchy lesions resembling those of an acute allergy)
- Tightened skin on the hands and feet
- Pigment loss or gain
- Calcium deposits in the skin. (They occur rather infrequently in people with lupus. They usually occur with inflammatory diseases of muscles, such as dermatomyositis or polymyositis.)
- Fluid-filled blisters
- Flat purple lesions

Which are the most common skin symptoms?

The discoid lesions, the blush rash, and the raised hives.

In general, what color are the rashes associated with lupus?

They tend to be red or purplish-blue.

What causes the facial rash in lupus?

It is generally caused by sun sensitivity.

Is this rash present all the time or only during a flare?

It is present after sun exposure and also during flares. (Although in some people sun exposure may cause flares, the facial rash can occur as a result of sun exposure even in those people who do not experience flares from sun sensitivity.) The rash can also redden after a period of fever or disease exacerbation. In some female patients, their rash occurs at certain times during their menstrual cycle. These events in some cases may or may not have anything to do with flares.

How do the rashes feel?

They can itch or burn. They may also ache and exude fluid like a blister. However, the vast majority of lupus rashes do not hurt at all.

What can be done about rashes?

Lupus rashes are particularly difficult to treat. Antiitch medications like antihistamines don't provide much relief. Painful rashes can be treated with topical anesthetics. Most rashes (especially the disfiguring ones) are treated with topical, or locally injected, steroids. In rare instances, it is necessary to use systemic steroids. The best systemic therapy, however, is the use of antimalarial drugs, which have recently come into favor because of their immunosuppressive effects, low toxicity, and mild anti-coagulant effects.

Does lupus cause the skin to peel?

Some people say that their skin does peel when they are experiencing symptoms of lupus. But this is not normally the case. Many arthritic diseases are associated with peeling skin of the palms of the hands and soles of the feet, but lupus is not one of them.

What causes hair loss (alopecia) in lupus? Is it permanent?

There can be many reasons for *alopecia,* none of which is certain (other than the use of certain medications—see the next question). Anyone going through hormonal changes can experience hair loss, such as women who have just given birth. However, both men and women with significantly severe lupus can lose their hair for reasons that aren't quite clear. The hair usually returns, so it is not considered permanent. Permanent hair loss all over the body can occur in association with lupus. This unusual condition is called *alopecia totalis.*

Which medications can cause hair loss in lupus?

Many medications cause hair loss, among them the widely used cytotoxic drugs like Cytoxan (cyclophosphamide) or Leukeran (chlorambucil). The drug Imuran (azathioprine) has also been known to produce hair loss. Most of these are reversible causes of hair loss.

Can lupus affect one's fingernails or toenails?

There are typical nail changes in lupus. Some lupus patients demonstrate a whitening and a scooping up of the end of the nail, which is called the *lupus nail*. This is probably due to a phenomenon called *onycholysis,* or the loosening of nails. At the present time, nothing can be done about this problem, other than generic lupus treatment.

Sometimes taking medications like Plaquenil (hydroxychloroquine sulfate) can change the color of nails to a darkish green color. Then there's another kind of nail change in which the nail develops lines across it. This change can be seen in many chronic diseases. In lupus, it most commonly is as a result of a chronic problem like kidney disease.

SUN SENSITIVITY

Are all lupus patients sun sensitive?

Approximately 35 to 50 percent of patients with lupus are sun sensitive. The reason that only some patients are sun sensitive is one of the great mysteries of this disease.

What causes sun sensitivity?

No one knows what happens when UV-B light comes into contact with the skin, or why it causes a worsening of systemic illness. It was originally thought that the sun damaged cells in the skin and these cells released DNA and other contents (such as RNA, RNP, glycoproteins, and other proteins), causing antigens from the cell to accumulate in the skin. However, this is still just a theory.

How does sun sensitivity affect an individual with lupus?

Sun sensitivity can be quite dangerous. Lupus patients should not go in the sun or be exposed to ultraviolet light. Exposed patients can suffer a terrible flare of the disease. They may develop signs of local disease in the skin such as rash, blisters, or redness with ulcerations. But even more serious is generalized disease due to sun sensitivity, which causes high fever, fatigue, and joint pains.

When do sun-related problems occur?

Usually within a few hours after sun exposure. Patients begin to suffer from joint pains, low-grade fever, and fatigue relatively quickly. These symptoms may or may not be accompanied by blistering; however, blistering does often occur in cases of extreme sensitivity.

Is there a difference in the effect of sun sensitivity in discoid lupus compared with its effects in SLE?

Both types of patients can be sun sensitive. Discoid patients are sometimes said to be more sun sensitive, but the potentially dangerous effects that are seen in patients with systemic lupus are not found in those with discoid lupus. Discoid lesions have immunoglobulin complexes deposited only in the actual lesions. It is believed that the lesions are definitely worsened by light exposure. Patients with SLE have deposits in skin both with lesions and without lesions.

What is the connection between ultraviolet light and lupus?

Ultraviolet light is the offending wavelength of light that causes the severe disease when one is sun sensitive. Ultraviolet light is divided into various wavelength ranges. The UV-A is not supposed to be dangerous to lupus patients at all. On the other hand, UV-B light is dangerous for patients with lupus who are sun sensitive.

Does sunlight or ultraviolet light cause lupus, or does it simply cause a flare of lupus?

Exposure to light does not cause lupus; it merely worsens the disease already present. However, until all the mechanisms of this disease are fully understood, we cannot know for sure.

Can fluorescent lights make lupus patients sick?

Some fluorescent lights emit UV-B and are therefore emitting light in the range that causes trouble. Therefore, lupus patients can be sensitive to fluorescent light, just as with sun sensitivity, and get sick.

What can be done to deal with sun sensitivity?

Limiting your exposure to the sun is the most effective way of dealing with sun sensitivity. When you must spend time in the sun, shield yourself from its rays. The use of hats, gloves, and long-sleeved dresses or shirts when outside is beneficial. Sunscreens are also very effective.

What sun protection factor (SPF) is usually recommended for individuals with lupus?

Select a sunscreen with an SPF of at least 15 to 30 or greater, depend-ing on the intensity of the sun and the amount of time you will be exposed to it.

Should sunblock be used all the time?

Because the sun's UV rays are always dangerous during the day, sunblock should be used at all times.

If one is sun sensitive, are there any times during the day when it's OK to go outside without protection?

Yes—at night! Even hazy or cloudy days produce enough sunlight to cause problems.

Does climatic change have any effect on the lupus sufferer?

Some data suggest that the change of seasons is associated with increased lupus flares. No one knows why this is so. It has something to do with a connection between light and the immune system, although most in-vestigators are still trying to figure out just what effect light has on the immune system.

KIDNEY COMPLICATIONS

What happens when lupus affects the kidneys?

As can happen with other organs, immune complexes can deposit in certain areas of the kidney. Their presence attracts white cells, which come and release certain kinds of chemicals that mediate inflammation and result in destruction of the kidney tissue. This is typical for all patients with lupus. However, more deposits of complexes with more damage is common in kidney failure. So there are varying degrees of severity. The patient would then need aggressive therapy (with powerful medications such as immunosuppressants, or with dialysis) or would risk succumbing to the disease.

What causes fluid retention in people with lupus?

Generally, the kidney has a remarkable ability to keep the body's fluids, solutes, and electrolytes in balance. The kidney can control the secretion and excretion of solutes and electrolytes. On the other hand, when the kidneys are not working properly, mineral balance is bad.

When you have lupus and you lose a lot of protein (which is one major solute in your kidneys), then you have less protein in your bloodstream than you have in your skin outside of the blood vessels. So the fluid tends to go where there is more solute. It leaves the blood vessels through the process of *osmosis* (the movement of fluid through a semipermeable membrane from an area of low concentration to an area of higher concentration) and accumulates under the skin, in the muscle fiber, and all over. This accumulation of fluid under the skin is known as *edema*.

Are there any other names for lupus of the kidneys?

There are several names for lupus of the kidneys, including *lupus nephritis, lupus nephrotic syndrome, immune complex nephritis,* and so on. In lupus, the kidneys can be affected by either the disease or the medication used to treat the disease. Some people refer to any kidney disease as renal or kidney failure. Kidney failure is the "end stage" of kidney disease.

What is nephrotic syndrome?

The membrane that supports filtration in the glomerulus (the filtering mechanism in the kidney that does all the filtering of the blood into urine) is called the *basement membrane.* When immune complexes or any other destructive complexes come along and create holes in the basement membrane, vital substances like proteins are lost. When this loss of proteins occurs, one is said to have *nephrotic syndrome.* The syndrome is not an acute process that can be treated aggressively with medications. Rather, nephrotic syndrome follows an acute phase of kidney disease. When it occurs, nephrotic syndrome is accompanied by high cholesterol, edema, and large amounts of protein in the urine.

Are all kidney problems in lupus nephritis problems?

Yes, nephritis means "inflammation of the kidney." Specifically, the patient has inflamed kidney tissue.

What percentage of lupus patients have kidney disease?

Approximately 75 percent of patients with lupus have some form of clinically significant kidney disease. There are many factors other than antibodies that predispose a person to kidney damage.

What factors predispose a person to kidney damage?

Beyond inflammation, destruction of the kidney can occur due to drugs like NSAIDs or to other forms of unrelated toxicity (like the deposition of chemicals or crystals in the kidney). For example, gout and the deposition of uric acid crystals in the kidney can result in the destruction of the kidneys, but gout and kidney stones in lupus patients are rare.

Why is kidney disease one of the worst complications of lupus?

Lupus kidney disease can be very dangerous. If not treated properly, toxins or poisons that would otherwise be filtered out from the blood by the kidneys can build up in the body, causing deteriorating physical condition and eventual death. Despite new understanding of the immune system and the recent aggressive use of chemotherapy to treat it, we have come no closer to preventing kidney disease. Without aggressive diagnosis and therapy, the patient's disease will progress, and kidney failure will be inevitable. However, most rheumatologists and nephrologists are often able to save the kidneys with aggressive early chemotherapy.

Are all kidney problems in lupus serious?

Some lesions are less serious than others. The severity of the kidney disease largely depends on the tissue-specific patterns of deposition. No one knows why the kidneys support this varied deposition, or why it occurs at all in some people and not in others. In fact, two people with the same apparent antibody types can have differences in the ways their kidneys are affected.

One form of the disease called *focal glomerulonephritis* is generally one of the less serious forms of kidney problems in lupus patients. Focal glomerulonephritis refers to small kidney lesions that are present in almost all patients with lupus. It means that there are small amounts of immune complexes deposited locally in the glomerulus of the kidney.

Membranoproliferative disease causes a much greater amount of protein to be lost in the urine. More serious than focal glomerulonephritis, membranoproliferative disease is still not as serious as *diffuse proliferative disease.*

Diffuse proliferative disease is the most severe form of the disease. It involves a lot of inflammation in the kidney because of greater amounts of deposition of immune complexes in the kidney, and it attracts a lot of white cells and other substances to cause inflammation. All forms of kidney disease in lupus patients must be carefully evaluated by a specialist and treated promptly.

How can someone with lupus tell when his or her kidney is affected?

Generally, swelling around the eyes or edema of the lower extremities suggests that kidney disease is present. Urine that is pink in color, along with sudden high blood pressure, headache, or a bloody nose can also suggest acute kidney disease.

How are doctors able to detect kidney problems?

When a doctor sees a lupus patient for the first time, a urinalysis should be performed and kidney function examined. A blood sample should also be taken. The laboratory technician looks for protein and unusual cells in the urine. If kidney failure is apparent, poisonous metabolites, like urea and other chemicals, are removed with either temporary (*intraperitoneal*) or permanent dialysis. Kidney failure is an emergency.

What is the purpose of twenty-four-hour urine collection?

Twenty-four-hour urine collection, required when the doctor discovers protein in the urine, can help make a quantitative assessment of the kidney's ability to excrete protein. The amount of protein in the urine can often tell the physician why the patient is swollen and give an estimate of kidney damage. Remember that loss of protein from the bloodstream into urine can result in movement of greater amounts of protein outside the blood vessels than inside. This results in the movement of fluid to the outside of the vessel, or edema. A twenty-four-hour urine collection also helps the doctor figure out the ability of the kidney to clear substances like *creatinine,* a waste produce of creatine metabolism. There are many calculations that help us understand kidney function based on weight of the patient, and so on, but none quite so helpful as the creatinine clearance, which is based on the filtration rate of the kidney.

What is the significance of blood in the urine?

Blood in the urine indicates that the red cells are passing into the urine from any number of sources, including the bladder, urethra, or the glomerulus (filtration mechanism) itself. It is usually a result of inflammation.

What is the significance of protein in the urine?

There are certain benign conditions that result in the appearance of small amounts of both protein and red cells in the urine. However, if the amount of protein is substantial, this can indicate a problem, such as kidney damage.

What type of blood tests are used to detect kidney failure?

Two major blood tests are used to test kidney functions—the tests for *blood urea nitrogen* (BUN) and *serum creatinine,* the breakdown products of protein metabolism. When these values rise, even slightly, there is cause for concern. This means that the kidneys are not working to remove the poisons that commonly accumulate in the body on a daily basis. The result can be uremia or poisoning of the body. This is kidney failure.

What are casts?

Casts are dead cells that retain the form of the tubules. When found in the urine, they indicate profound damage to the kidney. The appearance of white cell or red cell casts that have been eliminated from the kidney is, therefore, not a good sign.

What types of X-ray techniques are used with the kidney?

The simplest technique is the sonogram. It sizes the kidney and detects clots as a source of the protein in the urine or stones as a cause of pain. A renal vein thrombosis (clot in the renal vein) is often a major cause of protein in the urine and can be mistaken for nephrotic syndrome as a result of lupus if not detected with a sonogram.

Another major kidney exam (used in very special cases) is the *IVP* or *intravenous pyelogram*. In this procedure, dye is placed in the patient's system. An X-ray is then taken to see where the dye goes. This test is based on the timed excretion of dye from the urinary tract. It gives an indication of exactly how effective the excretion mechanisms are in a pair of kidneys.

The CAT scan and MRI have replaced most of the more complicated tests assessing renal function. These evaluate whether there are tumors or other space-occupying lesions like cysts and clots that may be causing the symptoms, rather than lupus.

When is it necessary for doctors to do a renal biopsy?

Once it is obvious that the patient is suffering from overt kidney disease as a result of lupus, a renal biopsy is usually performed. This is an invasive procedure that involves removing a piece of the kidney with a fine needle for examination. This is not always done without complications and therefore is done with caution. However, the biopsy is a good way of establishing not only the degree of acute versus chronic changes but also the pattern and extent of immune complex deposition. The kidney biopsy helps the doctor choose the right chemotherapy for a patient.

How is this procedure performed?

A needle is passed through the skin of the lower back. A piece of kidney tissue is obtained, which is placed in saline and sent to a laboratory for examination. The patient usually has to lie on his or her back after the procedure in order to be sure that no (or at least minimal) bleeding into the urinary tract or surrounding tissues occurs. The purpose of the biopsy is to look for the pathologic changes in the kidney that suggest damage. This is done by examining the *histology* (what the tissue looks like and how much damage has occurred) of the kidney lesion. During this process, we look at the tubules, glomerulus, and the rest of the tissue to see how it differs from normal kidney tissue. Sometimes the section of tissue is immunofluoresced to get a better picture of how much kidney damage has occurred as a result of autoimmune reaction.

What is the treatment for kidney problems?

There is no one fully accepted treatment for kidney problems. Most specialists use a combination of chemotherapeutic agents and sometimes corticosteroids for aggressive therapy of active lupus lesions. *Chemotherapy* refers to the use of poisonous agents (cytotoxic drugs). The drugs kill cells (both normal and abnormal). They are used to interrupt cell growth and therefore attempt to stop the growth of active lupus lesions that would otherwise have the potential to severely damage the kidneys.

What determines the level of medication therapy used for kidney complications?

This is often determined by the kidney biopsy. A rheumatologist and kidney expert get what is called an *activity and chronicity index* to determine whether there is enough activity in the kidney to justify the use of a potent chemotherapeutic agent. Such agents like Cytoxan and Imuran must never be used lightly.

What is the role of steroids in treatment of lupus nephritis?

If the lesions are minimal, and the results of the renal biopsy suggest something like membranoproliferative nephritis or focal glomerulonephritis, high-dose steroids might be used. In the case of severe disease, high-dose steroids and cytotoxic agents would be used. The steroids do not have to be administered orally. They can also be administered intravenously. *Pulse therapy* (brief, high doses of steroids) or large intravenous doses for short periods can be used to treat lupus nephritis. Pulse therapy allows the patient to receive very high doses of steroids over short periods of time. All of these therapies have side effects and must be used cautiously.

Steroids block many chemical pathways. They also stabilize the membranes in cells and prevent the release of inflammatory chemicals. Steroids also decrease the number of lymphocytes, or the cells that are specific to the immune system, in the blood. Ongoing research explores the immunosuppressive effects of steroids.

When are immunosuppressants used for lupus nephritis?

Immunosuppressants are used for most forms of lupus nephritis. However, they are not for everyone. The use of these agents depends on the nature of the lesion or the damage to the kidney. The renal lesion must show a fair degree of activity and low chronicity in order to justify use of such agents. Most forms of untreated lupus nephritis have activity and, therefore, require treatment. A biopsy will make this determination. A very acute lesion will respond to immunosuppressants more effectively than will a longer existing, more chronic one.

What is kidney failure?

Kidney failure is the total shutdown of kidney function. The kidneys can no longer filter urine or control what comes out in the urine. Inevitably, the patient cannot filter out the toxic products of metabolism, causing the BUN and the creatinine levels to rise, and the patient becomes ill. Generally, in lupus, this is a gradual process. However, it can progress relatively rapidly if the condition remains untreated. Most of the time, ignored symptoms like itching, nausea, easy bruising, and severe headache as a result of high blood pressure can be the result of almost total decline of kidney function. Without treatment, the patient will die.

How often do individuals with lupus experience kidney failure?

Fortunately, kidney failure does not occur in many lupus patients. However, almost 75 percent of all lupus patients will have suffered significant kidney damage as a result of their lupus. Much of the damage could possibly be prevented by early aggressive treatment with drugs.

Do all individuals with kidney failure require dialysis or transplantation?

Kidney failure is generally reversible—to a degree—if the process causing the kidney failure is stopped in its tracks. Therefore, few lupus patients in overt kidney failure require dialysis or transplants.

What is dialysis?

Dialysis is a method for removing poisons from the blood. It is used when the kidney can no longer perform this function itself.

What is involved in dialysis?

There are two kinds of dialysis. One is *peritoneal dialysis,* which utilizes the natural filtering mechanisms of the peritoneal membrane. A hole is made near the navel, and a tube is placed and sewn into the peritoneal cavity (the abdominal area, located in the belly where the intestines are situated). Fluid is exchanged through the peritoneum, exchanging the bad wastes for clean electrolyte-rich fluid. This process must be performed several hours per day in order to prevent uremia or uremic poisoning, which can be fatal.

A second form of dialysis is called *hemodialysis.* This procedure involves the attachment of a vascular shunt to a machine that filters the "bad" metabolites out of the circulation. This machine also uses a membrane (one that is very much like the peritoneal membrane but is synthetic) that allows the exchange of toxic metabolites.

Why do individuals on dialysis often experience improvement in their lupus?

No one knows for sure. Perhaps a substance involved in the cause of the disease is removed by the dialysis membrane. A curious aspect of dialysis, however, is the fact that many patients with lupus who undergo dialysis because of kidney failure have long-term remissions.

What is involved in kidney transplants?

A diseased kidney is replaced by a new one. However, this involves matching the new kidney. Kidney matching involves testing the genetic markers of the donor and recipient organs to make sure they are identical. This is done so that the new kidney is not rejected. In a body that daily rejects its own organs and tissues, a transplanted kidney is just another target to reject. Hence the use of immunosuppressants, which control the actual disease and allow the acceptance of the new, presumably "matched" kidney.

COMPLICATIONS OF THE NERVOUS SYSTEM

Lupus can affect both the peripheral nervous system and the central nervous system. What's the difference between these two systems?

Both are quite complex and affect function differently. The *peripheral nervous system* concerns itself with nerves that go to the extremities, or originate from the spinal cord. The spinal cord comes from the brain.

Anything outside the brain and spinal cord is part of the peripheral nervous system. The *central nervous system* is contained in the brain and the spinal cord.

What are the symptoms of peripheral and central nervous system complications?

Peripheral nervous system complications usually produce numbness and tingling and, later, overt weakness of a limb. In the central nervous system the symptoms can include anything from headache to coma. Central nervous system disease can also result in paralysis of a limb or several extremities, depending on where the lesion is located. Lesions in the brain due to central nervous system lupus can cause defective speech or vision and loss of sensation, temperature sense, and vibratory sense, among other effects.

What is lupus psychosis?

A severe behavioral abnormality that is a severe form of lupus of the brain, *lupus psychosis* causes the patient to behave very strangely and can result in significant disability. It is necessary to place lupus psychosis patients on medication to control their behavior. There do not seem to be any real physical changes in the brain to account for lupus psychosis. There may be chemical changes in the brain that are not visible on scans or other X-ray techniques.

Why is the nervous system affected by lupus?

As with any other tissue, the tissues of the nervous system can become a target antigen for lupus antibodies. When antibodies attack the brain, *cerebritis,* or inflammation of the brain, usually results. The flow of white cells and other debris-removing cells results in damage to the brain. Although temporary, this can cause significant disability. If scarring occurs, the damages can be permanent and leave a patient with lasting effects.

How often does lupus affect the peripheral nervous system?

Lupus affects the peripheral nervous system in less than 5 percent of lupus patients.

How often is the central nervous system affected in lupus?

Central nervous system complications in lupus are more common than originally thought. The brain is directly affected in about 25 percent of all cases. However, behavioral, or nonorganic, disease of the brain can occur in a much higher percentage (as high as 70 percent) of people with SLE.

Are there any other names for central nervous system lupus?

Yes. *Lupus psychosis* and *lupus cerebritis* are terms often used to refer to central nervous system lupus, although lupus psychosis implies a much *less* serious condition than lupus cerebritis. A patient who is diagnosed with true lupus cerebritis always requires chemotherapy. This is not the case with lupus psychosis, which could be caused by drugs used to treat the lupus as well as by the actual lupus. It is important to realize that lupus cerebritis can be the cause of lupus psychosis. This is one of the most difficult diagnoses for a doctor to make in patients with lupus.

What tests are used to detect problems in the brain?

There is no easy way to tell whether a patient has central nervous system lupus—not even with a brain biopsy. Several tests that are performed are a neurological clinical exam, a spinal tap for analysis of spinal fluid, possibly an electroencephalogram (EEG—a graphic record of electrical activity in the brain, through which doctors can determine the cause of seizure activity), and, more recently, a CAT scan or MRI, both of which are excellent at determining if any lesions exist in the brain.

Are there any tests used for peripheral nervous system complications?

There is only the clinical exam, which tests reflexes and sensation, including vibratory and temperature sense.

What is the treatment for nervous system complications?

Treatment is based on the symptoms being experienced (for example, antiseizure medications for seizures, and so on. Nevertheless, if the immune system is contributing to the neurological symptoms, then the patient needs to be treated with cytotoxic agents and other immunosuppressives, such as high doses of corticosteroids.

Is treatment for peripheral nervous system complications different from that for central nervous system problems?

No, treatment is the same.

Do people with lupus get many headaches?

Yes, and physicians are not sure why. They could be the result of some hormone or vascular change. Many lupus patients also get migraine headaches. Migraines are thought to be a result of disturbed *serotonin* (a transmitter in the brain) metabolism. Vascular headaches or migraines may also be the result of high blood pressure and should alert the patient to seek medical advice. These headaches usually occur in the back of the head and are often accompanied by a bloody nose. However, despite the fact that most headaches in lupus patients are of unknown cause, it *is* known that they are not life-threatening.

How are these headaches treated?

Severe headaches require a clinical exam. This includes a blood pressure check, an eye examination, a test of antibody levels, and perhaps even a spinal fluid analysis. Most headaches go away with Tylenol (acetaminophen) or aspirin. However, more severe headaches require other drugs such as potent prescription pain medications, vascular constrictors, or even immunosuppressive drugs (if the cause is deemed to be immunologically based).

Are fainting and blackouts common in lupus?

No. These are not routinely observed in lupus patients.

What causes people with lupus to have seizures?

Seizures are the result of lupus cerebritis. Increased or decreased electrical activity in the brain can be associated with seizure activity. This means that immune complex formation in the brain, leading to vasculitis and inflammation, is enough to cause cerebritis and seizures. Another possible cause is a small clot or an area of bleeding in the brain. All of these can be caused by lupus. There are, however, many other possible causes of seizure activity, and these must be ruled out before lupus can be determined to be the cause.

How can seizures be treated?

Seizures are often treated with sedative drugs like Valium (diazepam). The standard preventive measures for continued seizure activity include such drugs as Dilantin (phenytoin), Mysoline (primidone), Tegretol (carbamazepine), phenobarbital, and Depakote (divalproex sodium).

Are painful "pins and needles" in the palms of the hands a manifestation of lupus?

Pins and needles is not restricted to lupus. It can be caused by a variety of things. Generally, the extremities contain a variety of nerves that form what is called a dermatome, or pattern. Pins and needles in the palms of the hands might be the result of a neuropathy or may be part of a condition called carpal tunnel syndrome (a constriction over the median nerve in the wrist). Many patients with lupus have concurrent thyroid disease or diabetes and can thus develop these abnormalities.

What is the difference between organic and functional effect?

This is medical jargon. An organic effect indicates that the actual tissue of the brain is involved, whereas a functional effect is usually considered to be behavioral or psychological. Unfortunately, in many cases it is difficult to prove that functional effects are actually due to disease in tissue of the brain.

Why do many people with lupus experience memory problems?

Many people with lupus can experience significant memory problems, ranging from forgetfulness to memory loss. This may or may not be related to their medication doses or the activity of lupus itself. Although memory problems may be a frequent consequence of central nervous system lupus, some patients who do not have neuropsychiatric or central nervous system involvement can develop memory deficits (estimates are that approximately 40 percent of lupus patients who do not have central nervous system disease have deficits in short-term and/or long-term memory). The reasons for these deficits are not clear. These memory deficits are not related to emotional distress (although in some cases, this does play a role in further exacerbating memory problems), and the degree of memory problems may not correlate with the degree of disease activity. Therefore, it seems as though most impaired learning processes in lupus patients could be called residual, meaning they reflect dysfunction of the central nervous system due to the actual ravages of the disease on the rest of the body or to the possible prior or present use of medication (such as cortisone-like drugs).

What causes cognitive impairments other than memory loss, such as attention span or concentration difficulties in lupus patients?

There are a number of different cognitive abilities that may become impaired in those with lupus, such as the speed with which one processes thoughts, the ability to relate objects in time and space, and the way one processes emotions (or the way one feels about certain situations, which can be altered by the way one processes thoughts). It is not clear why these impairments exist. They may be due to specific antibody populations that may occur in patients with lupus. For example, people with a higher degree of cognitive impairment tend to have more antibodies to neurons than those who do not have cognitive impairment. Other areas being investigated include examining the shrinkage of certain parts of the brain due to certain drugs such as prednisone, cortisone, or some of the chemotherapeutic agents like Cytoxan (cyclophosphamide). These findings have only been reported in animals and have not yet been examined in humans.

Some studies have suggested a connection between lupus and learning disabilities such as dyslexia. How would that be explained?

These studies have not yet really explained this connection. They have only pointed out that there may be a connection. Earlier studies have shown that many patients with autoimmune diseases had learning disabilities. These patients often gave birth to children who were dyslexic and had variations in laterality (whether one does most of one's daily functions with the left or right side of the body) or loss of spatial relationship understanding and/or predominant left-handedness. In the mid-1980s, researchers in Boston found that patients with autoimmune disease of the thyroid gland or with certain inflammatory bowel diseases tended to be more likely to be left-handed or ambidextrous (able to use both hands equally). Eventually, studies were done with lupus patients, and while no significant increase in left-handedness or ambidexterity was found in patients with lupus, their children, specifically male children who did not have lupus, were found more often to be left-handed and have significantly more perceptual and learning disabilities such as dyslexia.

Many theories have been proposed to explain these findings (although none of them have been proven at this point). Some of them have focused on birth trauma, which is more common in offspring of lupus patients, the effects of antibodies on the developing baby's brain (an idea that has since been discounted), and last and most plausible, the effect of sex hormone changes in the mother on the developing brain in the fetus.

BLOOD COMPLICATIONS

What is the main blood problem for people with lupus?

Anemia. It is a lack of red blood cells or the presence of red blood cells that do not have enough oxygen-carrying capacity due to a deficiency in iron or vitamins. This occurs often in chronic illnesses. Iron or vitamin therapy can be effective with most forms of anemia. However, in the case of anemia of chronic lupus, neither iron nor vitamins are helpful in alleviating the condition.

How is anemia diagnosed?

The simplest way to diagnose anemia is to take a smear of the red blood cells and look at the cells under a microscope. This routine procedure will give an estimation of the size of the red cells, their density, and the intensity of redness (which is a reflection of the amount of hemoglobin in the cells).

What is hemolytic anemia?

"Hemolytic" means causing the disintegration of red blood cells. The red cells can be viewed as miniballoons carrying oxygen and hemoglobin. Antibodies are sometimes made against red cells. In the presence of other substances, like complement, these antibodies can pop the red cells; hence the term *hemolytic* anemia. Given enough time and the right amount of antibodies, the entire red cell population of the body eventually can be destroyed. This can be a very serious situation and must be treated early.

How is anemia treated?

Usually, treatment aims to reverse whatever caused the anemia in the first place. For example, if a patient is iron deficient, and the iron content in the body is replenished with iron supplements, the anemia goes away. In the chronic anemia of lupus, however, there is no treatment, at present, that is effective.

In hemolytic anemia, however, the offending agent is an antibody. The patient can take drugs, therefore, that will decrease the amount of antibody and reverse the anemic situation (prednisone, cortisone, or even cytotoxic agents are used in severe situations).

What is the significance of the lupus anticoagulant?

The lupus anticoagulant, ironically, *promotes* blood clotting. It is an antibody to phospholipid molecules that form the skeleton of the nerve cells, the heart valves, and most of the blood-clotting proteins. The lupus anticoagulant and/or antibodies to phospholipids can cause strokes, heart attacks, clots in the lung, blindness, and clots that cut off circulation to various organs.

What are some other blood problems?

Aside from anemia and lupus anticoagulants, antibodies against phospholipids like cardiolipin and other components of the blood like platelets are probably the causes of the most challenging of the lupus-related blood disorders. These will require many more years for full understanding.

What symptoms suggest the existence of blood problems?

In anemia, the symptoms are persistent headache, shortness of breath, and weakness. Patients with lupus anticoagulants, ironically, have problems with excessive clotting. A patient with phlebitis in a lower extremity (like the leg) or who experiences a sudden onset of chest pain and shortness of breath is probably experiencing clots. The shortness of breath is of significant concern because it might indicate a *pulmonary embolus* (a clot that blocks circulation to the lungs), which can be fatal.

A low platelet level indicates a condition called *thrombocytopenia*. This can cause significant bleeding, spontaneously and at any time, particularly if the platelets get below 10,000 (the normal platelet count is 150,000 to 300,000). Symptoms are usually bruising or easy bleeding.

How common are blood problems in lupus?

They are extremely common. Almost every lupus patient will develop anemia of chronic lupus. However, more severe anemia (such as hemolytic anemia) is present in less than 2 percent of patients. The lupus anticoagulant—although still under study in most patients—is found in over 35 percent of patients with the disease. Other phospholipid antibodies may be even more common. Anticardiolipin antibodies can be found in varying strength in over 80 percent of all lupus patients. They are the most commonly measured antibody against an entire group of phospholipids.

Why do many people with lupus experience a decrease in the number of white blood cells?

Low white cell count (known as *leukopenia*) is quite common in lupus patients and can often appear without symptoms. A patient is normally thought to have leukopenia if his or her white blood cell count falls to a level less than 3,000 (the normal white blood cell count is 5,000 to 10,000). This may suggest that a patient is about to experience a flare.

Antibodies can be made against any cell of the body in lupus patients. Polymorphonuclear (PMN) white cell antibodies attack all members of the white cell family. When the white cell count is decreased, it suggests that a patient is making antibodies toward the white cells as though they are germs, removing the white cells in organs like the spleen, and destroying them.

What is done about low white blood cell counts?

If a patient receives chemotherapy and has chemically lowered white cell counts, it is sometimes important to bring the white cell counts back to normal numbers in order to prevent infection or fever. This can be done by administering a chemical called a *cytokine,* which is normally produced by various immune cells and serves as a messenger to stimulate white cell growth and bring about a more effective immune response.

When a patient's white cell counts are low because of lupus, and the patient is undergoing a flare, it may be helpful or necessary to administer steroids like cortisone or prednisone to raise the level of white cells. Steroids release the white cells hanging around the walls of blood vessels, which increases the total white cell count.

Is a low white cell count as serious as the other blood disorders?

No. The lack of white cells or lymphocytes does not grossly affect the lupus patient unless the numbers become very low. For example, the lymphocytes of lupus patients never reach the low levels seen in AIDS patients, unless the patient has undergone chemotherapy, and the leukopenia would be a result of that. The loss of white blood cells has to be monitored, though, since white cell counts below a certain threshold may predispose the patient to infections that result in fever and/or sepsis (infection of the blood). When the white cell number becomes dangerously low, cytokines can reverse the process and increase the numbers of white cells.

Why is there often a decrease in the number of platelets in lupus?

Platelets most commonly disappear because of antiphospholipid antibodies, or because of antibodies against some other component on the surface of the platelet. A platelet can also be removed by the action of the spleen, in the case of *splenic engorgement*. (The spleen is the natural "end" of a platelet's life.)

What is done to treat the problem of low platelets?

Low platelets are generally increased by giving the patient prednisone. In other cases, the platelet numbers can actually be increased through chemotherapy with immunosuppressive drugs, which decreases the antibodies against the platelets. Generally, platelets have to be very low in lupus patients to warrant drug therapy. Patients with lupus are rarely given platelet infusions (a transfusion of platelets from another person) to raise the platelets because they usually make antibodies to the platelets (as they do with everything else). After new antiplatelet antibodies develop it would be nearly impossible to give the patient platelets again from any source.

What is ITP?

A disorder that can occur in both children and adults, *immune thrombocytopenic purpura (ITP)* is generally the result of antibodies toward platelets, which causes the platelet count to become very low. Patients with ITP have a tendency to bruise and bleed. When platelet levels are very low, spontaneous hemorrhaging can occur. In most people with low platelets, there are no symptoms, which makes this disorder very dangerous.

In severe cases, splenectomy, or removal of the spleen—the organ that removes the platelets from the blood—is generally the treatment of choice. Splenectomy is a common treatment for children, who generally have what is called acute ITP. In adults, the ITP is different. It is called chronic ITP. It is usually treated with drugs like Danazol, IVIG, and, sometimes, prednisone instead of the splenectomy. Sometimes it is absolutely necessary to remove the spleen, and many patients with lupus have had this done successfully.

Does everyone with ITP have lupus?

No. However, many lupus patients had ITP before their lupus was diagnosed. Some experts even believe that ITP is a precursor of lupus. It is more logical to assume that antiplatelet antibodies are part of the antiphospholipid group of antibodies since one of the major manifestations of antiphospholipid syndrome is low platelets. Apparently, antiphospholipid antibodies can stick to platelets and remove them. These antiplatelet antibodies are probably one of the earliest antibodies of lupus.

How often do people with lupus have blood transfusions?

A blood transfusion should never be given to a lupus patient unless absolutely necessary. Transfusions might result in the production of new antibodies against parts of the transfused blood that the immune system may recognize as antigens. In essence, one might form new antiplatelet antibodies or new red cell antibodies that had not previously existed. Dire situations that may require a lupus patient to receive a blood transfusion include gastrointestinal bleeding or severe trauma, such as a car accident.

COMPLICATIONS OF THE
CARDIOVASCULAR SYSTEM

What complications are related to the heart and circulatory system?

Problems related to circulation are high blood pressure (commonly found in the lupus patient with kidney disease) and pulmonary hypertension, or elevated blood pressure in the lungs, which can be extremely dangerous if not fatal.

The most serious diseases of the heart involve the valves. Vegetations (fibrin-rich materials that form and appear to get larger with time) can make the valves dysfunctional. Fortunately, this is not too common, and the increased use of the echocardiogram has made the detection of these vegetations easier. If these problems are found, valve replacement procedures can alleviate symptoms and signs of severe heart disease.

Actual disease of the conduction system of the heart (the electrical system of the heart that allows the heart to beat) is not too common in the adult with lupus but can be found in infants born to mothers with lupus who have the anti-Ro antibody. The conduction system of the heart thus becomes a target for this specific antibody, but only in newborns.

The phospholipid antibody has been associated with symptoms of increased pressure on the right side of the heart (pulmonary hypertension) and can be very dangerous to the patient. This condition can also occur in the absence of antibody and often requires that the patient receive a lung transplant.

Another condition is called *pericarditis,* or inflammation of the lining around the heart. It is a form of *serositis.* The problem that is most serious with this condition is the accumulation of fluid around the heart. This condition is called *cardiac tamponade.*

What is serositis?

Serosa are smooth membranes that line most of the organs in the body. *Serositis* is inflammation of the lining of organs. Since most organs of the body are lined with serosa, serositis can be a very painful and somewhat generalized condition.

How is it treated?

The ultimate therapy for conditions like serositis is immunosuppression, or the use of steroids or chemotherapeutic agents. However, since this is largely an inflammatory condition, the use of NSAIDs is often appropriate and may be enough by itself.

Why is bruising so common with lupus?

Bruising is a result of fragile blood vessels and low platelets or antibodies against phospholipids that cause bleeding under the skin. There can be antibodies against clotting factors and platelets because, among other things, these cells and factors contain phospholipids. The presence of these antibodies can cause clots to form or actually increase bleeding.

Bruising is most common, however, in patients who have been on steroids for a long time. Steroids cause the walls of the blood vessel to become somewhat fragile and allow the vessels—usually veins—to break with ease.

Are bruising problems dangerous?

Bruising problems are not dangerous unless they result in a massive collection of blood, which, if pressing on a vital avenue of circulation, can cause problems.

What is thrombophlebitis?

Thrombophlebitis is inflammation of the veins due to blood clots that occurs most commonly in the legs. The legs generally become swollen and red, which prevents the patient from walking easily. This can be quite dangerous, since the clots can break off and go to the lungs. The consequence of a clot that goes to the lungs (a *pulmonary embolus*) is difficulty breathing. This can actually result in death. Superficial thrombophlebitis, in which the affected veins are those just under the skin, is much less dangerous than deep vein thrombophlebitis.

What is vasculitis?

Vasculitis is an inflammation of the blood vessels. It can result in an abrupt cessation of circulation to a particular organ. Vasculitis of the bowel might result in a perforation of the bowel. Vasculitis of the brain might result in meningitis-like symptoms or actually cause coma. Vasculitis of the central nervous system might cause changes comparable to those of a stroke or cerebrovascular accident. Vasculitis can be reversed with chemotherapy or immunosuppression.

What is the difference between vasculitis and thrombophlebitis?

The inflammation in thrombophlebitis is due to a blood clot in the vessels. In addition, thrombophlebitis usually only affects the veins, whereas vasculitis can affect the veins and the arteries.

How often does vasculitis occur in lupus?

Vasculitis occurs with some frequency. Anywhere from 2 to 8 percent of patients with lupus have some form of vasculitis. An ongoing controversy at this time is whether phospholipid antibody syndrome causes vasculitis in patients.

Which blood vessels are affected by vasculitis?

All blood vessels can be affected by vasculitis. However, in lupus usually only the small to medium-sized veins and arteries are affected.

What causes vasculitis?

No one knows for sure. What *is* known is that when deposits of immune complexes are within the wall of a vessel, inflammation ensues, and an inflammatory reaction then compromises the vessel wall. Vasculitis can occur by itself or it can be associated with other diseases. There are many different forms such as lung vasculitis, brain vasculitis, and skin vasculitis. The most commonly associated diseases are lupus, rheumatoid arthritis, Sjogren's syndrome, and a condition known as hypersensitivity vasculitis, or vasculitis due to allergy.

What are the symptoms of vasculitis?

Often the only obvious symptoms of vasculitis are fever and weakness. If the vasculitis affects the skin, the symptoms include visible lesions. Vasculitis of other organs can cause inflammation and pain of the affected organ. Because vasculitis can be cryptic, happening insidiously and masquerading as something else, the affected organ can cease to function or be seriously damaged before the patient or the doctor even realizes that vasculitis is a problem. For example, vasculitis of the bowel can cause gastrointestinal bleeding, resulting in blood in the stool and severe abdominal pain. An entire bowel workup will reveal very little, except bleeding and abnormalities on angiography. Vasculitis is very difficult to diagnose.

How is vasculitis diagnosed?

With great difficulty! It is usually the last consideration in a diagnosis because it is fairly uncommon. X-ray changes of blood vessels observed after the injection of a dye and biopsies help to make a diagnosis. If the patient has serious lupus with many antibodies in the blood, it becomes much easier.

What determines which symptoms will occur?

This depends on which organs are affected and how extensively they are affected.

What is the most common type of vasculitis manifestation?

It is vasculitis of the skin because of the skin's large vascular, or blood vessel, makeup. If a person with lupus is going to have vasculitis, it will most probably be manifested in the skin.

What skin symptoms may indicate vasculitis?

Livedo reticulares, a condition characterized by a bluish "fishnet" appearance of the skin, is a common symptom of vasculitis. However, the appearance can vary. Ulcers or pustules are very common. Large purple bumps and small pinpoint hemorrhages can also be characteristic. Often the disease manifestation can be confirmed with a biopsy.

What are petechiae?

Petechiae are small hemorrhages, or pinpoint lesions, on the skin.

What are purpura?

Purpura are also raised hemorrhagic areas that are larger than petechiae and are somewhat purple in color.

What complications can occur as a result of vasculitis?

Infarction of an organ (lack of blood flow as a result of a narrowing or cutoff), irritation and inflammation (as in the case of the serous tissue surrounding the belly cavity or heart), generalized fever, and weakness are just a few possible vasculitis complications. If vasculitis occurs in the brain, an individual can become paralyzed on one side of the body or unable to speak (similar to a stroke).

What is the most serious form of vasculitis complication?

Vasculitis affecting the blood vessels of the central nervous system or the heart is the most serious complication.

How is vasculitis treated?

Large doses of immunosuppressants such as corticosteroids and/or chemotherapeutic agents like Cytoxan (cyclophosphamide) or Leukeran (chlorambucil) are used. Sometimes the vasculitis symptoms get better automatically when a flare of lupus is stopped or chemotherapy is instituted for other reasons, such as severe kidney or lung disease.

What is Raynaud's phenomenon?

It is a condition in which the blood vessels of the hands, feet, and other areas go into spasm. It is not known why this occurs.

Is it dangerous?

Raynaud's can result in the restriction or cessation of blood flow to a finger or toe or to the entire hand or foot. In extreme cases, it may cause gangrene or loss of an extremity.

What is the cause?

No one knows the causes of Raynaud's, other than that the spasms can be triggered by cold or stress.

What causes the skin to change color in Raynaud's?

The skin changes color because the flow of blood is either slowed or stopped in a blood vessel that narrows. On occasion the blood vessel can actually clog up, stopping the blood from flowing. The skin generally turns red, then white, and finally blue. A blue color indicates that there is no blood flow to the area. This a serious problem.

Why does Raynaud's affect mainly the extremities?

The extremities are most often affected because their blood vessels are small and often exposed to more extreme temperatures. However, there is some evidence that similar effects may occur in other areas such as the lung and intestine.

How is Raynaud's phenomenon treated?

The treatment of Raynaud's phenomenon has been the subject of many experimental investigations. Gravity may actually help. For example, shaking of arms or hands in a propeller motion can force blood flow to increase in the extremity. However, the usual manner in which Raynaud's is treated is by dilating the blood vessels using vasodilation drugs such as calcium channel-blocking drugs. Other drugs that cause vasodilation, such as topical nitroglycerin, are useful but limited due to other potential side effects. For example, extensive dilation of vessels may result in a sudden drop in blood pressure. Although this might help the Raynaud's, it can cause the patient to faint.

CHEST COMPLICATIONS

What percentage of lupus patients have chest problems?

Almost a third of patients with lupus have problems with their lungs, ranging from breathing abnormalities to pain or pressure upon breathing. Actual lupus pneumonitis must be distinguished from infection of the lung from immunosuppression, which is a very common problem.

What is pleurisy?

Pleurisy is a condition that is characterized by pain during breathing. The lungs are surrounded by sacs called *pleura*. When a patient breathes and these sacs rub against parts of the chest wall or the actual lung tissue, they become inflamed and cause pain.

What is pleuritis?

Pleuritis simply refers to this inflammation of the pleura.

What is the difference between pleurisy and pleuritis?

Pleurisy is mainly the pain produced by pleuritis.

What tests are used to check for pleurisy?

With the use of a stethoscope, a noise can often be heard that suggests that the lung lining may be rubbing against the chest wall, or some fluid might be present in the lung cavity, which may be the result of inflammation. A chest X-ray is also performed.

What is the treatment for pleurisy?

Generally, the inflammation is treated with anti-inflammatory drugs like aspirin or NSAIDs. Some physicians will also use steroids such as prednisone to treat pleurisy.

What is pericarditis?

Pericarditis is an inflammation of the lining of the heart or pericardium. The worst complication of this condition is pain in the chest, which can frighten you into believing you're having a heart attack. It can cause problems with the pump action of the heart. Since this pumping action can be impeded by fluid around the heart, the fluid must be inhibited or removed by suction with a fine needle.

Why does pericarditis sometimes feel like you're having a heart attack?

The pericardium has many nerve endings. When these become inflamed, it feels as though there is extreme pressure on the chest. Moreover, this pain can radiate to the left shoulder or arm, making the resemblance to a heart attack even greater.

How can you tell the difference?

You shouldn't even consider making a judgment about this by yourself. It could be *extremely* dangerous. Let your physician decide whether pericarditis is a possibility with a physical exam, electrocardiogram, and perhaps even with an echocardiogram.

How long does pericarditis usually last?

Pericarditis can last for a long time—as long as two weeks to two months, if not more.

What tests are used to detect pericarditis?

Again, the diagnosis can often be made with a stethoscope. The doctor looks for various sounds and signs when listening for pericarditis. A chest X-ray might be helpful. An electrocardiogram might also produce an unusual reading, and the fluid around the heart can "blunt" the electrical impulse and cause what is commonly referred to as "low voltage" in electrocardiography. This can confirm for the doctor that the patient has pericarditis.

How is pericarditis treated?

Because pericarditis is also an inflamed membrane, it can be treated with aspirin or NSAIDs. Prednisone is often used to inhibit the inflammatory process and prevent its recurrence; however, it is generally not used for long periods in this condition.

COMPLICATIONS OF THE DIGESTIVE SYSTEM

What are some complications of the digestive system?

Dyspepsia (gastric irritation), accompanied by pain and belching, is the most common symptom of gastric disease. The patient might also have significant nausea, especially on an empty stomach, and occasional (sometimes bloody) vomiting. These symptoms are very common in lupus. This is due largely to medication sometimes used as a lupus treatment that can stimulate gastric activity. Some of the pills given to patients for relief of joint pains or the cortisone taken to ameliorate the disease can cause severe gastritis and even gastric ulcers. Symptoms can include a pain in the middle region of the abdomen. Diarrhea, constipation, colitis (and rectal bleeding), and esophagus problems (inability to move food properly) are other symptoms that can be part of the gastrointestinal manifestations of lupus.

How are they diagnosed?

This is not always easy. The physician must rely on a careful history of the symptoms and signs of the disease. It is, therefore, important for the patient to provide an accurate and reliable history. Generally, tests for diagnosing problems in the gastrointestinal tract depend on the location and nature of the symptoms. Doctors often test liver or pancreatic function by checking for elevated liver- and/or pancreatic-derived chemicals in the blood, or they examine diseased areas directly with scopes to diagnose gastrointestinal problems.

How are digestive problems treated?

The treatment varies with the nature of the problem. The patient might require an antacid for relief of heartburn or medication to cause the muscle between the esophagus and stomach to relax. This treats the "heartburn," or the feeling that food is sticking in the throat. Often, directing the patient to abstain from eating for a determined period of time, coupled with antacids or acid receptor blockers, will help the patient's overall condition.

What symptoms are related to the intestinal tract?

The intestinal tract is responsible for the absorption of nutrients. Disorders of the intestinal tract can result in malabsorption, weight loss, poor blood clotting, constipation, or bloody diarrhea.

How are intestinal tract complications diagnosed?

Diagnosis is usually aided by the use of an *endoscope,* an instrument used to examine the inside of a hollow organ or body cavity. The doctor is able to cauterize bleeding areas, biopsy suspicious ones, and visualize and confirm problems right at the site, all with the use of the endoscope.

How are these problems treated?

Treatment often involves the use of agents that inhibit the secretion of acids in the intestinal tract. Antacids (tablets or liquids) can be useful for minor problems. For more serious problems, drugs that actually inhibit acid, like cimetidine (Tagamet) or ranitidine (Zantac), can be used. Newer drugs like omeprazole (Prilosec) can be very effective in decreasing stomach acid and healing ulcers.

What symptoms are related to the pancreas?

The pancreas makes enzymes for the digestion of food and fats, and it produces insulin, which is vital to the health of the body because it converts sugar in the body into energy. The reasons for recurrent *pancreatitis* (inflammation of the pancreas) in lupus are not clear, but it can be quite serious if not treated aggressively. Often a pancreatic *pseudocyst* (accumulations of tissue, fluid, blood, and other matter that are not true cysts because they do not have special cell linings) will result from such inflammation.

What symptoms are related to the liver?

The liver is usually not affected in patients with lupus unless they have active inflammation of the liver due to small vessel vasculitis. The major vessels of the liver can also be blocked with clots.

What is lupoid hepatitis?

Lupoid hepatitis is a liver disease that has no relationship to lupus. It just bears the name lupoid hepatitis (for reasons that are not clear). It is an autoimmune liver disease of young women. But it is not lupus.

How are liver and pancreas problems diagnosed?

Liver problems can be diagnosed through the use of simple blood tests, called liver function studies (LFTs). The doctor must determine whether or not the liver enzymes are elevated. Elevated liver enzymes would indicate the likelihood of abnormal liver functioning.

Pancreas problems are more difficult to diagnose. On most occasions of pancreatic problems, enzymes called amylase and lipase will become elevated. A sonogram (sound waves bounced off the abdomen) or other such scans can often aid in the diagnosis of pancreatic disease by detecting pseudocysts.

How are liver and pancreas problems treated?

The rare liver disease seen in lupus usually resolves itself. If an offending drug is the cause, then it is discontinued. Problems with the pancreas may also heal with time if no complications, such as bleeding and infection, exist. These problems require intense medical observation.

SYMPTOMS OF THE FEMALE REPRODUCTIVE SYSTEM

What is endometriosis, and what is the connection between it and lupus?

There is a definitive connection between endometriosis and lupus. Women with lupus have a higher incidence of endometriosis.

Women's uterine cells, which are normally eliminated monthly through the menstrual period, occasionally go in the reverse direction and come out the ends of the fallopian tubes into the stomach or the peritoneal cavity. When this happens, these cells are usually destroyed by the patient's immune system. A problem occurs in some women, however, when the cells persist and grow, in a way similar to a benign tumor. This is the disease known as *endometriosis*. The way to treat endometriosis is to administer a male hormone, such as Danocrine (danazol) or Lupron (leurolide acetate) that turns off the secretions of the pituitary gland, which stimulates hormone metabolism. When these drugs are given to a woman with endometriosis, the endometrial cells are destroyed.

Some women with endometriosis have rheumatic complaints that may often be confused with lupus. To confuse the matter of endometriosis and lupus more, women with endometriosis may have a lot of antibodies, specifically autoantibodies, such as antiphospholipid antibodies, and often a weakly positive ANA.

Is there a connection between ovarian cysts and lupus?

Recent studies have shown that women with lupus are more prone to ovarian cysts than women who do not have the disease. In fact, there are many women with so-called polycystic ovary disease, who, while they do not have lupus per se, have autoantibodies and intermittent joint pain that seem to occur at times of the year when their estrogen levels are the highest. These patients generally do not have menstrual periods, but they do have times during the year when their estrogen levels are higher than normal. Most of the findings of lupus occur when the estrogen levels are very high.

COMPLICATIONS OF THE MOUTH AND EYES

Why does lupus produce oral lesions?

Oral lesions, usually painful but sometimes painless, are thought to be caused by a form of vasculitis or inflammation of small blood vessels. These lesions are one of the best signals of lupus "flare."

Where in the mouth do they usually occur?

Most often they occur on the roof of the mouth. The painless lesions can usually only be detected by the physician.

What is Sjogren's syndrome?

Sjogren's syndrome (SjS) is an autoimmune disease that can be primary (occur by itself) but sometimes occurs with other autoimmune illnesses as well (secondary Sjogren's syndrome), including lupus. In SjS, the eyes, mouth, and other mucous membranes are dry. Tears, saliva, and vaginal fluids are scanty or absent, and the glands of the face (namely the parotids) are usually enlarged, possibly causing a "chipmunk-like" appearance. The dry mouth condition, called *xerostomia,* can result in dental caries due to the lack of protective enzymes contained in saliva. It is also called *sicca syndrome.*

What can be done about Sjogren's syndrome?

In general, SjS responds nicely to steroids like prednisone or cortisone. If symptoms aren't that severe, artificial saliva and tears are usually sufficient. Artificial saliva usually doesn't relieve any oral lesions that may be present, which can be very painful and can prevent the patient from eating. A local anesthetic, taken as a mouthwash, gargled, and sometimes even swallowed, can be helpful. Many new drugs, some of them derivatives of pilocarpine, are used to induce saliva and tears. Hydroxycellulose planchets, lubricating disks, can be placed under the eyelids to increase moisture. Secondary Sjogren's syndrome is not part of the typical case of lupus but is more often observed in rheumatoid arthritis.

What is antibiotic prophylaxis?

This means that antibiotics are administered, even if there is no actual infection. These are usually given to protect tissues or to prevent an infection when treatment of the mouth or bowels is undertaken. *Antibiotic prophylaxis* is an absolute necessity when there is a new heart murmur or proven vegetation on the valves. It is important to protect these protruding surfaces, which are subject to unusual currents of blood, from getting infected by passing bacteria. It is particularly difficult to remove and kill bacteria attached to heart valves or other areas that might be a resting place for invaders.

Does having lupus mean that one cannot be treated by a dentist?

No, all lupus patients should see a dentist regularly. Some dentists will consult a rheumatologist for advice. This is perfectly acceptable and even encouraged. For example, dentists might be concerned about bleeding in patients with clotting problems. Most patients with uncomplicated lupus do not require antibiotic prophylaxis during a dental procedure.

How can lupus affect the eyes?

Lupus normally has little effect on the eyes. But in rare cases, when problems do ensue, they may be devastating. For example, lupus can cause paralysis of the optic muscles that help the eyes to move, causing weakness. One can also have "cotton wool spots," or areas of vasculitis in the blood vessels of the eyes. Occlusions or blockages of the small vessels of the eyes rarely occur, but when they do, they can indicate the presence of phospholipid syndrome that can be caused by antiphospholipid antibodies. This syndrome is associated with the inappropriate clotting of blood in small or large blood vessels.

What are some of the symptoms of eye complications?

Double vision or actual loss of vision.

Does lupus result in an increased chance of glaucoma?

No.

Can lupus cause blindness?

Yes, but only in rare cases. For example, vision can be lost if small clots destroy the circulation in the retina (back of the eye). The nerves in the eye may also be affected by clots. The eye can have areas of vasculitis, which may cause bleeding into the eye. This is apt to be worse if the patient has antibodies against clotting factors or no platelets. When small blood vessels rupture or are inflamed, bleeding can occur. Any of these problems have the potential to cause blindness.

Cataracts caused by prolonged steroid use can also decrease vision, but this problem can be reversed surgically.

How are eye problems diagnosed?

Physicians examine the back of the eye with an ophthalmoscope. This should be done at the first visit and, certainly if there are vision complaints, during subsequent visits.

How can they be treated?

Anticoagulation (thinning of the blood), steroids, or even chemotherapy are appropriate treatments for lupus-caused vision problems. In cases where the eye is involved, your physician should consult with an ophthalmologist who is familiar with optic problems and lupus.

Can an individual with lupus wear contact lenses?

Yes, unless the patient has dry eyes and dry mouth symptoms.

INFECTIONS

Are individuals with lupus more prone to infections?

Lupus patients are not more prone to infections unless they are being treated for their lupus with immunosuppressants. Lupus patients who are being treated with immunosuppressive drugs have decreased immune function that makes them more susceptible to infection. They are prone to get opportunistic infections like molds and bacteria that under normal circumstances are not infective.

How are infections in people with lupus different from infections in other people?

Infections that occur in lupus patients being treated with immunosuppressive agents can be life-threatening since the body cannot fight off the infection. It is important to obtain rapid treatment with antibodies. Often the patient's white count is very depressed.

What tests are used to diagnose and evaluate infections?

Sometimes it is difficult to tell if a patient has an infection or if he or she is just experiencing a lupus flare. Tests of the C reactive protein (a nonspecific protein that rises and falls with certain illnesses and is low in lupus and elevated in infections) and the white blood count (also usually low in lupus but raised in patients with infection) are often used.

What is done to treat infections?

Patients are given *broad-spectrum* antibiotics, which usually cover a wide range of organisms, since there may not be enough time to establish which organism is responsible for weakness or high fever.

Should individuals with lupus be vaccinated?

Yes. Vaccination (immunization) does not increase the flare rates for lupus patients. Moreover, patients with *functional asplenia* (a dysfunction of the spleen due to immune complexes) may require a pneumococcal vaccine to protect against *streptococcus pneumoniae,* bacteria that are one of the most common causes of pneumonia.

Can lupus patients get the flu vaccine?

Yes, lupus patients are encouraged to get the flu vaccine by injection of the synthetic vaccine. Lupus patients should not get the nasal sprayed-live virus vaccine (FluMist).

Should lupus patients be immunized for smallpox?

No. Smallpox is a live virus vaccine. A patient who is immunosuppressed can become very ill when given a weakened smallpox vaccine.

Should lupus patients be vaccinated for hepatitis?

Again, lupus patients must be careful, but the hepatitis vaccine is usually based on a synthetic antigen. If the virus is not alive, lupus patients can receive it.

FATIGUE

What causes fatigue in lupus?

No one knows what causes fatigue in lupus. Despite the lack of information about fatigue in lupus, it is the most common complaint of lupus patients—perhaps one of the worst and most noncurable aspects of the disease. Even when you're treated, your antibodies are normal, and your disease is in remission, the fatigue can persist. Most often, it feels similar to a chronic case of the flu.

Some scientists believe that fatigue is the body's response to cytokines that are produced in many cells of the body. It is not known why the body responds this way or what the cytokines do to cause the body to respond by being fatigued. Research into these questions continues.

Is fatigue always physical, or can it also be psychological?

The feeling of fatigue is real. Feeling tired, drained, or exhausted is real. Fatigue can be due to lupus symptoms and the effects of lupus on the body. But in some cases, the fatigue may be partly psychological because of the way you feel emotionally, for example if you are depressed, bored, anxious, or just plain unhappy. There are some patients who, when told that they have a chronic illness, behave as they imagine a person would be expected to behave with a chronic illness. They may become highly dependent and gain other benefits by being fatigued. These are called *secondary gains* of illness. These secondary gains might be staying home from work or school with an excuse or getting out of doing household chores. They now have an excuse for being fatigued because they have the label *lupus,* and they use that excuse.

What can be done about fatigue?

There are no specific medical treatments currently that can improve fatigue. There are several drugs in development that appear to have some success in battling fatigue. There include male hormones. The way the male hormones probably work is to inhibit certain cytokines and therefore reduce the fatigue. Some patients claim that treatment with corticosteroids helps. Others find relief with newer drugs like anabolic steroids. However, it is unlikely that an overall effective treatment will be found until we better understand the cause of the disease.

Certainly one of the things that's important in dealing with fatigue is to rest. Fatigue is the body's way of saying that it needs rest. Rest may be the only thing that can really help fatigue. (See chapter 4 for more about rest and exercise.)

PAIN

Why is lupus such a painful disease?

This is due to inflammation in the body.

How many people with lupus experience pain?

All lupus patients experience pain. The immune complexes that form in lupus cause varying degrees of pain and discomfort. This is due largely to the release of inflammatory mediators like histamine and serotonin when the cells respond to the areas of immune attack.

How does stress contribute to pain?

Stress causes a tensing of muscles, both increasing pain and making it more difficult to relax.

How does fatigue contribute to pain?

Fatigue does not allow tissues and joints to get the rest they need to repair themselves. This can contribute to the overall pain experienced.

How does depression contribute to pain?

When patients are depressed, they tend to be less active. As such, they have more time to think about how they are feeling. Hence their awareness of their pain can be heightened.

What kinds of treatment can be useful in treating pain?

There are four traditional categories of treatment for pain: chemical (the use of medication to destroy or block the chemical transmission of pain down the nerve fibers), surgical (cutting the nerves, thus preventing transmission of the electrical impulse), physical (the use of physical therapy procedures such as exercise, hot/cold, and so on to send different messages to the brain), and psychological (teaching one to deal more effectively with the pain by using coping strategies or by substituting some other feeling for the pain, thus distracting attention from the pain). In general, all four treatments work by interrupting the transmission of pain messages before the brain receives and interprets them.

Many books, programs, and techniques give information on how to reduce pain. A number of beneficial books are listed in the appendix, and some of the most helpful techniques, such as physical therapy, are explained in chapter 4.

Does psychological treatment for pain imply that "pain is all in one's head"?

No. Although pain is physiological, the perception of it can be exacerbated by psychological interpretation. Techniques involved in pain control can actually reduce the perception of pain and therefore the discomfort caused by it. For example, relaxation techniques, which can reduce stress or tension, can also reduce the impact of pain.

Relaxation techniques are widely accepted as being effective techniques for patient self-improvement programs to deal not only with pain but with virtually any aspect of living with lupus. Books giving more information about relaxation techniques are listed in the appendix.

What are the most commonly prescribed pain medications for lupus?

Pain medication is useful for lupus. However, it is very common to become addicted to it, especially when more powerful narcotics are used. So pain medication should be used with discretion.

The most common pain medications for lupus can be either analgesic, which numb the actual pain, or anti-inflammatory, which decrease the pain by decreasing pain-causing inflammation. Analgesics include Tylenol (acetaminophen) and drugs like Darvon (propoxyphene hydrochloride). Anti-inflammatory drugs include Advil and Motrin (ibuprofen). In more extreme cases, pain can be treated with such narcotic preparations as Percocet or Percodan (oxycodone), Demerol (meperidine hydrochloride), or even morphine sulfate.

COMPLICATIONS OF THE BLOOD

What is the phospholipid syndrome?

The phospholipid syndrome causes the blood to be in a *procoagulant state,* a state in which the blood becomes very sticky and has a tendency to clot. It can coexist with lupus or occur by itself. This syndrome is characterized by the occurrence of a number of the antibodies against various clotting factors and other proteins (antiphospholipid antibodies). It is usually associated with clots, miscarriages, and low platelets. People with phospholipid syndrome often have to go on anticoagulants, which can either be natural or synthetic drugs.

Do all lupus patients have antiphospholipid syndrome?

No, only about 40 percent of lupus patients have the antiphospholipid antibodies. Many patients with these antibodies will never clot, but these antibodies may also have an important role in high blood pressure and accelerated atherosclerosis.

What are the phospholipids?

The phospholipids are fats that have phosphate groups on them. Phospholipids make up most cell membranes, are part of molecules like clotting factors, and often form the structural aspects of heart valves and parts of the human brain. Phospholipids float around in the blood with proteins in order to balance the electrical charges of phospholipid molecules.

What is an antiphospholipid?

An antiphospholipid is an antibody directed against the phospholipid molecule that occurs only during autoimmunity. Since autoimmunity is a natural process of the body, antiphospholipid antibodies have been found in those without autoimmune disease. It is also found in diabetics, people with severe infections, HIV patients, those with strokes, pregnant women, and those with lupus.

It is possible that antiphospholipid activates the clotting system in blood vessels within the body. Most commonly, clotting can cause the obstruction of one or more small blood vessels such as the retinal artery or a vessel in the upper extremity, but clots can be deadly. One of the most common causes of death is pulmonary embolus, which can occur in a patient with antiphospholipid syndrome.

What is anticardiolipin?

Cardiolipin is one form of phospholipid, but to many doctors cardiolipin and phospholipid are synonymous. Cardiolipin is found in the heart valves, the inner parts of our cells, and makes up the inner parts of bacteria called *spirochetes*. One such spirochete is the syphilis organism.

What is the false positive syphilis test?

A false positive syphilis test is a test that is positive in the absence of the actual disease syphilis. It is often found in patients with antiphospholipid antibodies.

What is the antiphospholipid brain connection?

An MRI often reveals that patients who have antiphospholipid syndrome have areas in the brain that look like demyelination has occurred. Demyelination is the removal of the covering of the nerve. Myelin is like insulation of the nerve, and its removal results in disturbed transmission. It is often difficult in patients to differentiate the phospholipid syndrome from multiple sclerosis or Lyme disease. Patients with the antiphospholipid brain lesions often have symptoms of multiple sclerosis, such as numbness in the fingers and toes and dizziness. Some require specific tests for multiple sclerosis such as a spinal tap or visual evoked responses to make the differentiation.

What specific tests help diagnose antiphospholipid syndrome?

There are many. The most common test is a simple PT with a PTT. In the phospholipid syndrome the PTT is often elevated, meaning that the patient's blood fails to clot in the test tube. This is the so-called lupus inhibitor. Lupus anticoagulant is really not an anticoagulant at all but rather a substance that enhances the clotting of blood. More specific tests should include anticardiolipin antibodies of the IgG, IgM, and anti IgA variety. Sometimes a physician may look for an antibody to a protein called the beta 2 glycoprotein-1.

What is beta 2 glycoprotein-1?

This is a protein that, attached to the phospholipid, allows it to travel within the blood freely. Some feel that this protein is the true target of the antiphospholipid antibody. This protein is also called apolipoprotein H; it is a natural anticoagulant.

What are some of the tests that determine the presence of a lupus anticoagulant?

The best and cheapest test to help you find a lupus anticoagulant is the PTT. However, there are many ways to find this complex. They include the Russell viper venom time (RVVT), the Kaolin clotting test, and others.

What medicines do I take if I never had a clot?

If you have never had a clot but just have the abnormal tests, you probably do not need any medication. Some doctors will give the patient baby aspirin, which is a good idea for everyone because it helps prevent stroke and heart attacks by preventing the clumping of platelets.

What medicines do I take if I already have had a clot?

If you have had a clot and have antibodies to the phospholipid proteins, then you must be on anticoagulation medication for the rest of your life.

What is heparin?

Heparin is a blood thinner that prevents clotting and is often given to patients by injection to keep the blood thin after a clot has formed. This is a drug, but it is also made by certain cells of the body. The anticlotting activity of heparin has to be monitored by a physician.

Low-molecular-weight heparin is a drug that is derived from the chemical breakdown of regular-sized heparin. The low-molecular-weight heparin does not have to be monitored like regular heparin, and it has some different properties. Heparin can cause platelets to disappear and bone to be reabsorbed when used over a long period of time. For this reason the low-molecular-weight heparin is preferred when possible.

What is Coumadin?

This drug acts on vitamin K–dependent proteins in the blood to prevent clotting. It is also known as warfarin and rat poison because it kills animals like rats by preventing their blood from clotting. Because it acts on vitamin-dependent clotting factors, diet and other drugs may affect its potency. Coumadin measures the prothrombin time (PT) to determine something called INR (international normalized ratio), which is the standard measure to determine the efficiency of blood thinning. The normal INR is usually around 1.0. When you are taking Coumadin your INR is elevated and should be at 3.0 to 3.5.

If Coumadin is not regulated, blood may become thin, causing excessive bleeding. Some INRs can go very high, and you can bleed spontaneously. Often diet, other drugs, and overall metabolic changes can cause the INR to go out of range. This is why it is important to have the INR measured with frequency when you are taking Coumadin. Some doctors feel that the INR should be measured weekly or biweekly if you are taking Coumadin.

4.

TREATMENT OF LUPUS

I n all probability, your most important questions about lupus involve its treatment. You'll want to know everything you can about what can be done to treat the disease. Since there is no cure for lupus, the goal of treatment is symptom suppression and, it is hoped, remission (elimination of symptoms). There are a number of different modalities (types, categories, or methods) of treatment for lupus. This chapter will provide answers to questions about many of these modalities, other than medication, which will be discussed in chapter 5.

SOME GENERAL INFORMATION

What is the general goal of treatment for lupus?

The goal is to prevent the immune system from attacking and destroying vital organs.

Q Does everybody with lupus
    require treatment?

No, treatment is not required at all times. However, almost all lupus patients will probably require some type of treatment at some point or another. This must be determined by the doctor on an individual basis.

Q Are there any treatments that are used
    only with adults, not children?

There is usually no difference in the use of drugs in adults and children, except in the dosage. A doctor might be reluctant to use potent drugs such as immunosuppressants on a child because of possible side effects, including limitations on growth and, later, fertility.

Q Are any treatments used with children
    that are not used with adults?

No.

Q Do treatments differ, depending
    on the physician?

Yes. Physicians may interpret a finding differently. Some physicians might be more aggressive than others. However, life-threatening conditions are usually treated in the same way.

Why do different physicians sometimes prescribe different treatments for the same patient?

Different treatments can sometimes achieve the same effect. For example, one physician might wish to immunosuppress a patient with cortisone, while another might choose to use Cytoxan (cyclophosphamide). It is a matter of choice for both the doctor and patient. The patient, of course, has the right to question anything of which she or he is unsure.

How often should individuals with lupus see the doctor?

This depends on the severity of the disease and the way it affects the body. Some patients have little significant organ damage while others have a more aggressive form of the disease. Some patients might be asked to return weekly, while others may require a checkup once a month (or even less often when experiencing no effects).

What is done during normal follow-up visits to the doctor?

The most important aspect of the physical examination is the history. During the initial diagnostic appointments, the history obtains all relevant medical information about the patient. During followup visits, the history is extended to obtain information about everything that has happened since the last appointment. It is very important that the patient tell the doctor everything that is bothering him or her. By asking the right questions, it becomes easier for the physician to accurately monitor the course of lupus, determining which changes in treatment may be necessitated by the course of the disease.

A physical examination is then completed. The physical examination is performed to determine whether there's anything wrong with various parts of the body. Then blood is drawn to test the antibody and complement values, which determine how active the disease is and whether or not the disease is changing direction, and, consequently, whether or not the treatment should be changed.

Why is it important for individuals with lupus to have their blood tested regularly?

Most often, blood tests are used to predict a lupus flare. In addition, total dosages of prednisone or other drugs may be altered on the basis of test results. In some rare instances, the tests might indicate a serious yet nonobvious condition.

Why is it important for people with lupus to be aware of quackery?

Quackery is the intentional promotion or use of ineffective drugs or remedies. Since lupus is not yet curable, there is a great potential for fraudulent or criminal activity regarding the treatment of it. People have been known to make fortunes off patients with chronic illnesses who desperately spend a lot of money for less-than-appropriate "remedies."

How can quackery hurt me physically?

Occasionally, a substance that is prescribed can actually worsen your illness.

How can lupus patients protect themselves from quackery?

Only medications approved by the Food and Drug Administration and prescribed or recommended by a competent and legitimate physician should be used. This will ensure that you are not taking anything that could be harmful to your health.

TREATMENT MODALITIES

What role does physical therapy play in lupus treatment?

Physical therapy (PT) can play a large role in lupus treatment. For patients who have a great deal of pain and require bed rest, physical therapy helps to keep the muscles limber. It can also keep them strong and relaxed and can relieve stress. Aerobic exercise is the most important form of physical therapy. Although physical therapy is normally designed for patients who have limited mobility after injury, exercise can also be helpful for individuals with lupus.

Do all lupus patients require physical therapy?

Lupus patients who are in the acute phase of their illnesses should not get physical therapy since it can make the disease worse. But someone who is not acutely ill, is not suffering from a flare, and whose deformity or weakness is not very severe can benefit from PT. It is also recommended for patients who have contractures, bad osteoporosis, neurological weakness, and joint deformities as a result of lupus or its treatment.

How beneficial is physical therapy in treating pain?

Physical therapy does not treat pain, but it may provide some psychological relief.

Can physical therapy help improve joint pain?

Lupus joint pain will not respond to physical therapy, since the mechanisms of lupus pain are different from that of physical injury. However, as mentioned earlier, physical therapy can be used to remobilize patients after a long period of bed rest.

What is the role of heat and cold in treatment of pain?

Heat and cold can provide topical relief of pain and inflammation after an injury. They might also be of some use in cases of severe inflammation. In lupus, however, only medication is useful as a way of treating or reversing inflammation. Hot and cold can provide some soothing relief, but that's the extent of its benefits.

What is plasmapheresis?

Plasmapheresis is the removal and cleansing of the blood. Most antibodies and proteins are present in the noncellular part of the blood or plasma. This plasma can be removed by machine and later replaced by different plasma. Because the current method of cleansing plasma is ineffective, it is difficult, except under experimental conditions, to wash the patient's plasma (remove the antibodies) and then return it to the patient.

When is plasmapheresis used?

Doctors have not had much success in treating lupus patients with plasmapheresis. However, it is currently being used as a lupus treatment in Germany with chemotherapy, with somewhat promising results. In lupus, the antibodies that are removed from the plasma return very quickly. Hence the patient would need to be plasmapheresed frequently (for example, every other day). This is not without risk. Moreover, there is no proof that enough antibody is removed to prevent later problems.

What are the dangers in plasmapheresis?

Since the patient is attached to a machine for about three hours, there is always the danger of bleeding or infection. Moreover, there must be easy access to large veins. This becomes more and more difficult over time because the blood vessels can only handle a few holes poked into them, and a fairly large needle is used. Too many holes will cause a lot of hemorrhaging and bruising. As a result, as with dialysis patients, shunts (artificial connectors in the blood vessels) have to be put in the veins because you can't keep sticking needles in the same blood vessel.

What are the similarities between dialysis and plasmapheresis?

There are many. Toxic materials are being removed through the use of a machine in both processes. In dialysis, the components removed are small toxic chemicals, such as urea nitrogen, creatinine, and potassium, that can build up and poison the body. In plasmapheresis, the substances removed are larger proteins. In dialysis, the blood goes through membranes that filter the poisonous material from it, and then the blood returns to the body. In plasmapheresis, however, the substances are too big for this process, so instead of being cleansed, the plasma is completely removed and replaced.

Can acupuncture be helpful in treating pain?

Acupuncture has been used successfully to treat pain, particularly in other countries, like China.

Can chiropractic techniques be helpful?

Chiropractic techniques are good for adjusting bones and relieving pressure on muscles. In lupus, however, there is an immunologically based pathology in joints and muscles. Chiropractic is not going to cure the disease, but it might be helpful in certain cases, under the proper medical supervision, in making the patient feel more comfortable.

What is the role of biofeedback in pain treatment?

Biofeedback is a method in which the patient learns to alter certain body functions, such as blood pressure, with the use of electronic monitoring of changes in body function. It has been used to reduce pain in certain symptoms of lupus such as Raynaud's phenomenon. Unfortunately, however, there is little data to scientifically support its use.

What is the role of psychotherapy, or counseling?

Psychotherapy, or counseling, helps patients to verbalize and work through any feelings of denial, anger, fear, or frustration about their impairments and limitations. It is very helpful in guiding patients to learn methods of coping with their illness and to gain a sense of control by using preventive measures. In addition, counseling can help patients to see their accomplishments despite any limitations.

What is alternative medicine?

Alternative medicine is the use of techniques outside of traditional medicine. Examples of alternative medicine include acupuncture, homeopathy, herbal medicine, massage therapy, chiropractic methods, yoga, biofeedback, and hypnosis. Many of these techniques can also be helpful in relieving insomnia, chronic pain, stress, and headaches.

What is the role of homeopathic and/or herbal remedies in treatment of lupus?

Homeopathy is a treatment system based on the use of small doses of a drug that in large doses would actually cause the symptoms that are being treated. Herbal medicine is the use of natural herbs to promote healing. There is little scientific data to support the use of these alternative therapies.

Is there any danger in combining traditional Western drug therapy with nontraditional remedies?

Yes. Many drugs, foods, and herbs do not mix well. One of these may negate the other, or they may have an adverse chemical reaction.

DIET AND WEIGHT CHANGES

Does diet play a role in lupus treatment?

While it is important to have a nutritionally sound diet, it does not seem to play a significant role in the treatment of general lupus, though there are certain cases in which dietary modifications may be helpful. Research is exploring this area. Work with your physician to determine which, if any, modifications might be helpful in your case.

What types of dietary modifications might be helpful?

Foods low in fat and lots of vegetables can be helpful. One area of research deals with a chemical called indole-3-carbinol that may be very good for you. It is present in certain kinds of cruciferous vegetables, including kale, cabbage, and Brussels sprouts.

If the kidneys are affected by lupus, is dietary intervention necessary?

Yes, dietary intervention is mandatory for people with severe kidney disease. It may be necessary to limit protein intake for someone with kidney failure because the end products of protein metabolism cause the buildup of toxic chemicals such as urea nitrogen, uric acid, and potassium. Since the kidney's filtering capabilities are diminished with kidney disease, there's more of a chance of the body being poisoned. In the case of high blood pressure and edema, it is usually necessary to limit the patient's salt intake and perhaps even fluid intake. These recommendations cannot be generalized. They are specific for each person.

Should caffeine be limited or avoided?

No, there is no reason to limit or avoid caffeine because of lupus.

What should be done about fat and cholesterol in one's diet?

These can be lowered voluntarily. However, it should be known that patients on steroids will have higher fat levels in their blood. This also applies to people with kidney disease. The full significance of fats in the blood of lupus patients is not known at present. It is known, however, that people with very high cholesterol are at considerable risk for heart pathology and should take conscious steps to lower dietary fat.

How appropriate is a high-fiber diet?

A diet high in fiber is good for almost anybody, not just people with lupus.

How necessary is it to take vitamin supplements?

This is a good idea. People with lupus often become debilitated and do not get enough nutrients. Even though most physicians believe that a balanced diet ensures getting enough vitamins, it's probably still a good idea to take vitamin supplements, particularly during an illness.

Can people with lupus take cod liver oil since it contains vitamin D?

Yes, patients can take vitamin D–containing substances with mineral supplements like calcium. Their bones can certainly benefit from such supplements.

Is it true that the immune response to some foods may stimulate or exacerbate episodes of lupus?

There is no evidence of this in humans, but some lab mice with lupus have become ill upon exposure to milk proteins. A form of drug-induced lupus has been found in monkeys fed huge amounts of alfalfa sprouts.

How often do people with lupus become overweight?

People with lupus very frequently gain weight, especially after steroid treatment, because the steroids cause deposition of fat in unusual areas and fluid and salt retention, and they increase the appetite. Such weight gain is usually reversible. It is always healthier to try to maintain a normal weight.

What can or should be done about weight changes?

Consulting your physician is a good start. Most can tell whether you need additional testing or clinical investigation regarding your weight.

REST AND EXERCISE

Why is it important to get enough rest?

One form of therapy for mild to moderate lupus is bed rest. The body needs time to heal itself. There is an old theory that overactivity and exhaustion lead to a release of "self" antigens, which can perpetuate a flare. Rest is very good for both body and mind.

How much rest is required?

A patient with lupus should have at least seven hours of solid sleep per night. This rest will help the patient to feel refreshed. Too little rest can lead to a flare.

Why is exercise important?

Exercise is very important for normal muscle function and to maintain integrity of the bones. It is vital that patients with lupus do not feel that they are useless or unable to exercise. Some patients cease to function entirely and even rely on the assistance of wheelchairs. Most patients with lupus are capable of some type of exercise to increase the aerobic capacity of cells and improve immune function.

How does exercise help the body?

There is no body system that does not benefit from good exercise. Exercise can build and maintain muscle tone, support and stabilize joints, reduce fatigue, and maintain or increase mobility. Exercise is also good for the mind. (Of course, one does not want to overdo it!)

How often should you exercise?

Many factors are involved in determining how often you should exercise and what exercises you should do. Because there are so many variables involved, the best advice is to consult your physician.

Are there times when you shouldn't exercise?

Definitely! Whenever you are having a flare, exercise becomes dangerous and unwise. Bed rest is absolutely necessary. Achy muscles and a feeling of total exhaustion will usually indicate that you are incapable of exercising at this time.

What type of exercise is most appropriate for people with lupus?

Aerobic conditioning exercise.

What types of exercise should be avoided?

Isometric exercises are to be used with caution. These exercises involve tensing of the muscles, which causes the release of large amounts of auto-antigen. Directly exercising the muscles releases nucleic acids and a variety of other proteins into the blood. If you have lupus, it is believed that exposing your immune system to such proteins causes it to react even more strongly to reexposure. This will make you sick.

What are passive range of motion (ROM) exercises?

These involve moving an arm or leg with assistance. Passive means that you don't put any of your own energy or motor skill into the movement. This movement is, instead, provided by someone else.

What is the difference between passive ROM and active-assistive ROM?

Active-assistive ROM is motion that *you* initiate, even though you're being assisted with the motion by someone or something else.

NONMEDICAL THERAPY OF LUPUS

. . . .

Medicine is not the only way to treat lupus and its symptoms. Following is a summary of the nonmedical therapies that are effective as treatments for lupus.

- Good diet and nutrition
- Lots of rest
- Lots of exercise (doctor's approval needed)
- Avoiding the sun if you are sun sensitive
- Adjustment of your work schedule to be as stress-free as possible
- Avoiding allergic attacks if you have allergies, which are more common in lupus patients

When are these exercises appropriate for lupus?

Both passive and active-assistive ROM exercises can be helpful when there has been disuse, damage, or injury to an extremity, and movement cannot be done on your own.

5.

MEDICATION

. . . .

Medication is the primary medical treatment for lupus. There are a number of different medications, of various potencies and with various uses, that can play a role in lupus treatment. This chapter provides answers for questions about the use of medication, including which are the most frequently used medications, why each medication is used, what each one does, and what possible side effects may occur.

MEDICATION OVERVIEW

Why is medication one of the most important components of treatment for lupus?

Medication is the *only way* to treat *severe* lupus. At the present time, there are no other methods available to treat lupus because there is nothing else that can have the necessary impact on the immune system.

What is the basic goal of drug treatment for lupus?

The goal is to weaken the immune system so that the large number of antibodies and cells that attack a person's body are minimal or no longer present.

Why is prescribing medication always such a trial-and-error process?

Every patient is different. Some patients have very active immune systems. Others have immune systems that are not so active. But the immune system is not the only factor. Each patient reacts to each drug differently. You could give the exact same medication to five people and get five different responses.

There are probably many factors that determine how well a medication will work, including age, hormonal status, systems and symptoms involved, and even the diet of the patient. Severity of the disease is also important. For example, someone with lupus that is particularly life-threatening may require a formula of several immunosuppressives, rather than just one drug. All of this—and more—must be considered when prescribing medication.

Do all medications have side effects?

They usually do. Some side effects are more serious than others, and when severe enough, the offending drug may have to be discontinued. Other side effects are minor and can be diminished by altering the dosage.

Are side effects reversible?

They usually are. This is true even when the white blood cell count has been drastically reduced through the use of chemotherapeutic agents.

However, one example of an irreversible side effect, even when medication is stopped, is the death of bone (*avascular necrosis*) from drugs like cortisone. In these cases, surgery may be necessary as one way to correct the situation.

Why is it important to keep clear records of the drugs I am taking?

All drugs have the potential for side effects and to interact with other drugs. Over-the-counter medications and even vitamins should be noted by your physician. Nothing that goes in your body should be neglected. Special diets, liquid or otherwise, should also be noted for your record.

Are any of the drugs commonly prescribed for lupus dangerous in their interactions?

The drugs used to treat lupus can be dangerous in their potency. In the case of lupus, inexperienced doctors can overtreat patients. But for the most part, drugs that are given to lupus patients do not interact with each other negatively. Drugs can have a cumulative effect and make each other stronger if used improperly, however.

Why is the goal of treatment to get the person off the medication?

Drugs are not healthy for anyone, including lupus patients. With lupus, drugs are being used to either suppress the immune system or get rid of inflammation. Doctors aim to accomplish these goals as soon as possible, and then take the patient off the medication. No one should be on medication any longer than is necessary.

ASPIRIN

What is aspirin?

Aspirin is an anti-inflammatory, antipyretic (fever-reducing), analgesic agent. Its clinical name is acetylsalicylic acid.

How does aspirin work in the treatment of lupus?

Aspirin works as an analgesic (pain-reliever) by working on the central nervous system and reducing your ability to feel pain. It also reduces the low-grade fevers that frequently occur in lupus. At higher dosages, aspirin works as an anti-inflammatory drug by blocking the production of inflammation-triggering prostaglandins.

Why is aspirin used?

Aspirin inhibits, and often reverses, the inflammatory process. It works by decreasing inflammation generally and locally. It inhibits certain enzymes and chemical mediators of inflammation, such as the prostaglandins. These are very important chemicals in the inflammatory process. They can be both protective and harmful to body tissues. Aspirin stops the cells from going to the site of the injury and secreting the chemicals that cause inflammation.

Why is it important to lower fever in someone with lupus?

It's not medically important to lower fever in lupus because the fever is usually low grade (usually below 100° F). Fever reduction with aspirin is usually done for the patient's comfort.

What dosage of aspirin is appropriate?

In most diseases, like rheumatoid arthritis, the dosage of aspirin can be raised very high. Ringing in the ears (or tinnitus) indicates that a patient has reached his or her limit in dosage. However, in lupus, the case is different. High dosages of aspirin can cause significant kidney and liver problems. Therefore, aspirin dosages for patients with lupus should probably be limited to no more than eight per day, or four every six hours.

What are the side effects of using aspirin?

When aspirin inhibits the prostaglandins that coat the stomach, small ulcers form, and pain and bleeding in the stools ensue. Some people's stomachs are very sensitive to the effects of aspirin. Side effects also include liver enzyme abnormalities and a decrease in blood flow to the kidneys. Ringing in the ears can occur at higher dosages.

What can be done about these side effects?

Nothing. Most go away when the aspirin intake is stopped or the dosage is decreased.

What is the difference between Tylenol and aspirin?

Tylenol is *acetaminophen*. While it, too, has analgesic and antipyretic properties, Tylenol is not an anti-inflammatory drug. Both aspirin and Tylenol can be used to treat pain and to lower body temperature.

If Tylenol is used, what dosage is appropriate?

Two tablets every four to six hours is adequate. Caution should be taken, however, since some serious side effects, like liver or kidney disease, can occur with misuse of this drug.

NSAIDS (NONSTEROIDAL ANTI-INFLAMMATORY DRUGS)

What are NSAIDs?

NSAIDs are a class of drugs that are stronger than aspirin that are used to control inflammation and pain without steroids. NSAIDs inhibit the production of either the COX-1 or COX-2 enzyme or both. The COX-1 enzyme is involved in the production of prostaglandins that protect the stomach. COX-2 enzymes are involved in the production of prostaglandins that promote pain, fever, and inflammation. NSAIDs are most commonly prescribed for joint pains, muscle pains, and feelings of general discomfort. COX-1 may also prevent blood clots—but not to the degree that aspirin does.

NSAIDs that block the COX-1 enzyme (either alone or in combination with COX-2 enzymes) have the side effect of causing damage to the stomach lining, often resulting in GI upset, ulcers, and bleeding. Drugs that only inhibit the COX-2 enzyme reduce the chance of bleeding or stomach upset when taking them, but bleeding can still occur if they are not monitored. Stomach upset is the most common side effect of NSAIDs.

Can I take NSAIDs for lupus?

COX-2 inhibitors can relieve the pain and inflammation associated with lupus for some people. However, more serious side effects can occur for those with severe lupus or reduced kidney function, as NSAIDs may decrease the filtration of blood through the kidney and make the blood urea nitrogen and serum creatine levels rise, resulting in kidney failure. All people taking COX inhibitor drugs or NSAIDs should be careful about their kidneys. Lupus patients are at special risk because many have compromised kidney function already. NSAIDs can also raise blood pressure.

There are at least twenty types of NSAIDs available that act in different ways within the body. Some doctors may try several to see which formulation works best for a particular patient. Doses of NSAIDs vary with the brand, and some have potentially dangerous side effects due to their potency. NSAIDs act on symptoms, rather than the cause of the disease. They should not be used for serious complications of lupus like kidney, lung, skin, or brain disease.

ANTIMALARIALS

What are antimalarials?

Antimalarials are broad-spectrum, antiinfective agents that were originally developed to prevent a person from becoming infected with the malarial parasite. They have mild immunosuppressive properties and can be taken for long periods of time. They also lower blood cholesterol and act as mild anticoagulants.

When are antimalarials suggested in lupus treatment?

Since they are mild immunosuppressants, antimalarials can be used in most forms of mild lupus. They can also be beneficial in more serious forms of the disease, if accompanied by stronger drugs like prednisone to treat symptoms that are not helped by the antimalarials alone.

Why is prednisone often prescribed with antimalarials?

There are times when doctors may not get the desired results using only antimalarials. They may then decide to add prednisone to the treatment. Prednisone does not enhance the effects of antimalarials. Rather, the combination of the two drugs will better treat the symptoms being experienced.

Are antimalarials used to try to help patients get off prednisone?

Sometimes. Antimalarial drugs are milder than prednisone. If the antimalarial works, and the prednisone dosage can be weaned down to a very manageable dose, then the goal is to manage the disease with the antimalarial by itself.

Is it true that there are cases where antimalarials and prednisone continue to be used together to bring about different effects?

Yes. Let's take an example. Plaquenil (hydroxychloroquine sulfate) is an antimalarial that is very good for skin lupus. Plaquenil may be used by some doctors to control the size of skin lesions and to indirectly control hair growth, which is lost in areas around lupus skin lesions. Prednisone cannot always be as effective in this area as an antimalarial. Some doctors decide, once they introduce prednisone, to stop the Plaquenil. Others continue to use prednisone with antimalarials because the little extra kick of immunosuppression from the antimalarials can sometimes help in keeping the dosage of prednisone lower than it might otherwise have to be, which can minimize or reduce the likelihood of the side effects that might come from the higher dosages of prednisone.

What are the most commonly used antimalarials?

Plaquenil (hydroxychloroquine sulfate) and *Aralen* (chloroquine).

How long does it take for these drugs to work?

Anywhere from three to six weeks.

Can antimalarials be used in combination with other drugs?

Yes. In fact, they are most commonly used in combination with other drugs because antimalarials are mild drugs, and some symptoms may require other drugs to treat them. As these symptoms become controlled and no longer require the other medications, the antimalarial drugs can be used by themselves.

What side effects can occur with antimalarials?

Common side effects are nausea and rash. Less common but more serious side effects are vision problems, such as *retinal degeneration* (the rods and cones behind the eye degenerate and pigment is deposited there) and *corneal anesthesia* (the surface of the eye loses feeling). Most of the time these effects are reversible as long as the drug is stopped early. However, permanent vision loss has been reported due to these effects. These side effects can appear at any time during the course of therapy. However, they are most common within two months after starting the drug.

Q Is it important for someone taking antimalarials
    to have regular eye examinations?

Yes. Any visual complaints must be brought to the attention of a physician immediately. Immediate eye examinations can prevent future blindness.

Q How often should these eye examinations
    take place?

According to the *Physician's Desk Reference,* which provides facts about all prescribed medications, those taking antimalarials should have their eyes examined every six months.

Q What can be done about the side effects
    of antimalarials?

Nothing, except stopping the drugs.

CORTICOSTEROIDS

Q What are corticosteroids?

Corticosteroids are the chemicals commonly known as steroids. They are normally produced by the cortex of the adrenal gland, which sits atop the kidneys and produces many chemicals. Corticosteroids, like the other chemicals secreted by the adrenal gland, give extra strength and power to the body in times of need. Corticosteroids are among the most powerful and frequently used drugs in the treatment of lupus.

What are some other names for corticosteroids?

Corticosteroids are also referred to as *glucocorticoids, cortisones,* or *prednisone.*

How are corticosteroids produced?

They are synthesized in, and secreted by, the adrenal gland.

What are the most commonly used corticosteroids?

The most commonly used corticosteroid in lupus is prednisone. Other commonly used corticosteroids are *prednisolone,* which is chemically changed for easy passage through the liver; *hydrocortisone,* which is weaker in strength than prednisone; *methylprednisolone,* which is stronger than prednisone; and *Decadron* (dexamethasone) which is extremely potent and used only in unusual circumstances.

Are corticosteroids a type of anti-inflammatory?

The corticosteroids are the strongest known anti-inflammatory drugs. There is still much controversy as to what the actual anti-inflammatory actions of these drugs are, but they are known to decrease cytokines (mediators of inflammation) by preventing their manufacture and release; stabilize the inflammatory mediators contained in the compartments of cellular particles called endosomes so that they will not trigger more of an inflammatory reaction; and actually kill cells or delay the synthesis of other inflammatory chemicals.

How are corticosteroids administered?

They are given orally whenever possible. However, in certain cases they are given intravenously. Intravenous administration may be used in severe disease or when you want to give the patient a high dose very quickly but eliminate the side effects. Sometimes they are even injected directly into an inflamed area, such as the joint space.

What is the difference between corticosteroids in the form of pills and topical steroid creams or ointments?

The major difference between pills and ointments is that the ointments are absorbed locally into the inflamed skin, usually for a rash or local lesion. There are usually fewer systemic side effects with topical creams. However, if used in great concentration on the skin, the patient may suffer all the side effects of the drug, just as if he or she were taking it orally or intravenously. Patients who take the pills experience major side effects if the drug is taken for a long period of time.

What are the side effects of corticosteroids?

There are many. The most significant ones are the *Cushing effects* (named after the surgeon who first described them), accumulation of fat in unusual areas, such as over the spine and stomach; thinning of the skin; easy bruising; resorption of bones (osteoporosis); cataracts; depression; and steroid psychosis.

When do physicians usually decide to use corticosteroids in treatment?

Corticosteroids are used when the immune system requires something stronger than anti-inflammatories like NSAIDs to suppress it, or to control potentially dangerous symptoms that are otherwise not being controlled. Corticosteroids are generally used for the more severe manifestations of lupus, not when symptoms can be controlled with other kinds of drugs, such as NSAIDs.

How do corticosteroids affect the adrenal glands?

Steroids are endocrine hormones. As such, they suppress the body's own natural production of these hormones. When cortisone is given, the adrenal gland suppresses its own synthesis and secretion of cortisone. This is a negative effect. If the steroid is given for a long time, the adrenal gland will actually atrophy or grow smaller.

What are the typical dosages of corticosteroids?

There is no typical dosage. However, it is generally believed that any dosage over 20 milligrams per day will result in some adrenal atrophy if given over a long period of time. This dosage is approximately equal to the daily physiological secretion of hormone from the adrenal gland. As a result, the adrenal glands will no longer need to produce cortisone, and the pills will consequently replace the naturally secreted hormone.

Some patients never want to get off cortisone. Cortisone is an essential stress hormone and, as such, is needed for the normal workings of the body. In other words, it prepares you for action. It makes you feel strong and can create a feeling of euphoria. Some people believe that they're able to get more done when they're on higher levels of steroids.

It is not addictive, but it does make patients feel good. When you are no longer taking cortisone, you don't feel as good as you did when you were taking it. Small dosages of the drug are generally useful for a short period of time but should not be used for many years because of the side effects.

What are considered to be low, moderate, and high dosages of corticosteroids?

A low dosage of corticosteroids is anything below 10 milligrams per day, a moderate dosage would be around 30 milligrams, and 60 milligrams or above per day is considered high. These figures are based on dosages of prednisone. It is important to know that 5 milligrams of prednisone is approximately equivalent to 25 milligrams of cortisone.

Why is it so important to comply with my corticosteroid prescription?

The function of the adrenal gland—a gland essential for life because it produces key hormones that regulate salt and water metabolism, and is the source of adrenaline, the "fight or flight" hormone—is inhibited by large dosages of corticosteroids and "turns off" when they are administered. The gland can recover, but it needs time. Therefore, stopping the drug suddenly results in no cortisone in the body. This can be life-threatening. Most patients get very ill if they mistakenly stop their cortisone therapy abruptly.

Why is it so important to reduce prednisone dosages gradually?

When one reduces the prednisone dosage gradually, the adrenal gland gradually returns to full function. Once full function returns, the drug can be completely discontinued. Some individuals who have not been on the drug for very long (usually less than one month), or who have tapered off with sufficient care that their adrenal gland is back to normal, can come off the drug completely.

What is a typical taper schedule for cortisone?

Cortisone must be tapered because the adrenal gland has been inhibited from making natural cortisone for the period of time that you take the drug. The cortisone that comes from the adrenal gland is very important to body function, and if you do not retrain the adrenal gland to produce its own cortisone, you run the risk of being deficient in cortisone, resulting in a condition called Addison's disease. An example of a typical taper schedule is lowering the dosage of cortisone every other day or gradually decreasing the dose daily. The length of time a patient has been on the drug and the amount of stress the patient is under are important factors the doctor should consider when determining the tapering schedule.

What is the alternate-day treatment strategy?

With alternate-day treatment, instead of taking cortisone every day, the patient takes corticosteroids every other day (or, in some cases, the patient takes different amounts of corticosteroids on alternate days).

Why is alternate-day treatment used?

By giving the patient an "every other day" dosage, the gland is never really allowed to stop secreting on its own. Tapering off the drug occurs more effectively (and less traumatically) than if the drug were dropped abruptly or reduced from an every-day strategy. This may help the adrenal gland to resume complete functioning more quickly when the patient comes off corticosteroids. It is also believed that alternate-day treatment minimizes the potential side effects.

What is pulse therapy?

Pulse therapy (also known as *bolus therapy*) involves the administration of large amounts of corticosteroids over a short period of time, such as three hours. It is believed that the use of large dosages (1,000 milligrams at a time) can have a much more powerful effect on the body than small ones. Various pulse regimes exist, such as monthly three-day therapy sessions with one gram (1,000 milligrams) being given at each session.

When is pulse therapy used?

It may be used during a severe lupus flare, or in cases where there is danger to significant organs (like severe kidney or brain disease).

Does pulse therapy always work?

No, not always. It is just another attempt at treating lupus. In some patients, the side effects of pulse therapy can be even worse than the disease itself.

What are some of these negative effects of pulse therapy?

Seizures, an initial superficial rise in the results of kidney function tests (such as the BUN and the creatinine), high blood pressure, and extremely high levels of blood sugar may result. Because of the possibility of these side effects, pulse therapy usually requires a hospital stay, although it occasionally can be done at home in the presence of a nurse or a doctor.

What causes swelling due to corticosteroids?

Corticosteroids regulate salt metabolism and may cause the retention of salts and, consequently, the retention of fluids. This can cause swelling. It can also be caused by the accumulation of fat that is common with steroid treatment.

Why do corticosteroids sometimes cause hair growth?

Cortisone has an androgenic, or male hormone, effect. For this reason, it can cause hair growth and acne. This effect, although troublesome, is less serious than some of the other side effects of corticosteroids.

Why do some individuals taking corticosteroids gain weight?

Steroids cause the deposition of fat in unusual areas, and salt and fluid retention, which cause weight gain. They also increase the appetite, which, of course, also contributes to weight gain.

What is osteoporosis, and what causes it in individuals with lupus?

Osteoporosis is the resorption or loss of calcium from bones. The bones become thin and much weaker. Corticosteroids can cause or accelerate osteoporosis. Osteoporosis that occurs in lupus patients who aren't taking corticosteroids is caused by inactivity, such as prolonged bed rest.

Is it helpful for individuals on corticosteroids to take calcium supplements?

Yes. People with osteoporosis are encouraged to take calcium daily and vitamin D once a week, if needed. Some doctors recommend supplemental fluoride and even male and female hormones, but what benefits these supplements may bring is still controversial. Other agents are used to treat osteoporosis, such as bisphosphonates, synthetic substances that are believed to coat the bone surface and prevent disintegration, and calcitonin, a thyroid gland hormone that regulates calcium metabolism and prevents the disintegration of bone. Doctors generally obtain a measure of bone density before starting the use of these agents.

Some doctors believe that an individual being treated with corticosteroids should take calcium supplements before osteoporosis even develops. Others feel that it won't make much of a difference. Discuss this with your doctor.

How do calcium supplements help?

They provide the building blocks for the osteoblasts, cells that help to place the calcium in the bone itself.

What dosage of calcium is most appropriate?

Most excess calcium is excreted. It is generally believed that people who eat well get enough natural calcium in foods. However, in patients who are losing calcium due to corticosteroids, supplemental calcium is a good idea. Although the recommended dosage depends on many factors, it usually ranges anywhere from 600 to 1,500 milligrams per day, depending on your doctor.

Can anything be done about osteoporosis?

Prevention is the best recommendation at this time. The best way to prevent osteoporosis depends on who you are. For example, if you're a young woman who has had her ovaries removed, and your source of estrogen is gone, you may need estrogen replacement therapy. Caution is warranted, however, in lupus patients because estrogen may exacerbate their lupus. Researchers are examining the safety issue of estrogen therapy in postmenopausal lupus patients. In general, the best ways to try to prevent osteoporosis are through activity, exercise, and a good diet complete with calcium and vitamin D.

Treatment of osteoporosis today is quite sophisticated, and many new agents exist that are effective to some degree. Much current research is exploring more effective ways to treat osteoporosis. For example, new agents that have been approved include Miacalcin (calcitonin), which can be taken either by injection or as a nasal spray, and the bisphosphonates, which include drugs such as Fosamax (alendronate).

Why do many patients on corticosteroids develop cataracts?

Cortisone is one of the few hormones that can spontaneously bind to proteins like the collagen in a lens. The cortisone "caramelizes" on the lens, which results in the clouding we know as *cataracts*.

What is done to treat cataracts?

Since the formation of a cataract is irreversible, removing the lens and replacing it with another one is necessary.

What is avascular necrosis, and why does it occur in individuals on corticosteriods?

Avascular necrosis is the death of bone due to lack of circulation to that particular area. A current theory is that because corticosteroids raise the level of fat in the blood, small fat plugs form in small arterioles of the long bones and actually obstruct the flow of blood to the bone.

What exactly happens to the bone in avascular necrosis?

The healthy bone requires nourishing with oxygen and nutrients. It gets this from blood circulation. If the bone's blood supply is cut off, causing what is called an infarct (an area of dead tissue due to lack of circulation), it does not receive the necessary nutrients, and that segment of bone dies. It loses its strength and structure, and a cavity can form, often because of a loss of calcium. Eventually there will be actual collapse of the bone.

What body parts are most affected by avascular necrosis?

The hip bones are the most commonly affected. The long bones in the legs and arms, like the femur and humerus, are also often affected. However, in some patients, all long bones are affected.

What is the difference between ischemic necrosis, avascular necrosis, and aseptic necrosis?

These are different terms for the same condition.

What is the exact cause of avascular necrosis?

No one knows. There is considerable evidence that it may occur in people with lupus who have not even taken corticosteroids. However, most experts feel that the vast majority of cases are a result of corticosteroids.

How is avascular necrosis treated?

Treatment requires removal of the segment of dead bone. If the dead segment is part of a joint, the entire joint might be replaced with an artificial prosthesis.

How often is this surgery necessary?

Surgery is necessary in about 60 percent of cases.

What is done to help individuals who experience depression or other psychogenic disturbances when using corticosteroids?

Some people can experience depression or other emotional problems as a result of using corticosteroids. It is important for a professional to distinguish whether or not these psychogenic disturbances are due to corticosteroids, because if the depression or other disturbances are severe, the corticosteroids must be stopped and replaced with a substitute immunosuppressive agent such as Imuran (azathioprine) or other cytotoxic drugs.

Q Can prolonged use of corticosteroids damage the kidneys?

No. However, related side effects such as high blood pressure or high blood sugar as a result of corticosteroid use might damage the kidneys.

IMMUNOSUPPRESSANTS

Q What are immunosuppressive or cytotoxic drugs?

Immunosuppressive or *cytotoxic drugs* suppress immune function. They can suppress any arm of the immune system, like T cells or B cells. They can even suppress transplanted organ rejection; the making of antibodies; or the attack of certain cells, viruses, or tumors.

Q If cytotoxic drugs and corticosteroids are both immunosuppressive, then what's the difference between them?

This is like comparing apples and oranges. They both accomplish the same end; however, getting to the end varies with each agent. Chemotherapy, or the use of cytotoxic drugs, usually results in some sort of effects quickly. The drugs are given quickly, and they act with speed. Corticosteroids also act quickly but do not have the drastic, irreversible effects of a poison. The goal is the same: to weaken the immune system so that antibody and toxic cells are not directed to the body's other cells and tissues.

Are cytotoxic drugs considered poison?

Yes. They are toxic. They are killers of cells. That's what *cytotoxic* means.

Why is the use of these drugs sometimes referred to as chemotherapy?

Most people think of anticancer agents when they think of chemotherapy. However, all chemical substances used to treat disease are chemotherapeutic.

How can immunosuppressants be helpful in lupus treatment?

These drugs can inhibit the abnormal or "hyper-" immune response.

How do immunosuppressants work?

They kill or inhibit the action of the immune system. This can result in the death of cells or the interruption of the synthesis of antibody. Remember that certain cells of the immune system manufacture antibodies. These antibodies are very important in lupus. They are the proteins that combine with an antigen or foreign substance. In the case of lupus, the antigens are "self" proteins or molecules. Thus, if we turn off the manufacture of the antibodies, the damage done to the body, as a result of immune complexes, ceases.

What immunosuppressives are used in lupus treatment?

Some agents that are classically referred to as chemotherapy include Cytoxan, Imuran, Leukeran, and Rheumatrex or methotrexate. Newer agents include CellCept and rituximab.

What are some of the chronic changes?

The biggest concern for patients on chemo is the later development of a malignancy like a lymphoma or other form of blood disease. Sometimes this happens twenty years after taking the chemo drug, and no one can be absolutely sure that the chemo is responsible in all cases. However, these are manageable in most cases and should be easily detected for treatment by your doctor.

When are immunosuppressives used?

These drugs are reserved for the treatment of very serious diseases like deterioration of kidney function or lung or heart disease. They are not drugs of last resort, but rather very potent agents that can achieve a fair amount of success at low dosages.

What exactly do they do?

The chemotherapy agents regulate the making of antibody and the total populations of cells that react against yourself. Each drug has different actions, depending on its nature. For example, Cytoxan (cyclophosphamide) is an alkylating agent. *Alkylating agents* are basically chemicals that "interrupt" growth of cells by placing alkyl chemical groups in the DNA molecules to prevent them from being read or transcribed by the cell. If the information in the DNA molecules cannot be read or transcribed, they can't make proteins or grow or reproduce. Imuran (azathioprine) is changed in the body to another type of alkylating agent. Again, the ultimate effect is to interrupt the cell cycle.

What are the primary side effects of using immunosuppressive drugs?

Their effects can be very serious and life-threatening. While these drugs are helpful because they stop cell growth as immunosuppressants, they can also be harmful because they can ruin normal tissues. Generally, the cells of the body that divide the quickest are the ones that are poisoned the earliest and, as such, are also inhibited, along with the "bad" cells that are targeted. Examples of fast-growing cells that can be affected include those in the bone marrow, the gums, the hair follicles, and the cells of the bowel wall. The cells of the bowel wall are the most rapidly dividing cells of the body, and death of these cells poses the biggest problems. This can lead to serious diarrhea and increasing difficulty absorbing food.

Right after the chemotherapy, you can have a drop of your white count, fever, hair loss, blisters in your mouth, and a variety of other changes. Fortunately, this does not happen to everyone, and it is usually short-lived. Surprisingly, the biggest complaints after chemotherapy are nausea and hair loss. The hair will come back, and the nausea is transient and can be treated by drugs.

What complications can arise with the use of immunosuppressants?

Possible complications include bone marrow suppression, hair loss, ulcers in the mouth and stomach, liver disease (like hepatitis), and bleeding disorders. But these are all uncommon if the administration of the drug is monitored by a specialist.

How can these complications
be best dealt with?

Often the toxic effects of drugs can be prevented by taking counter-measures. In the case of Cytoxan (cyclophosphamide), for example, one must drink a lot of fluids. This keeps the metabolites from the Cytoxan—which are toxic to the bladder—out of the bladder so they can do very little harm. It keeps them diluted and reduces the chances of bladder irritation and bleeding. There are also drugs that can be given to patients that will minimize the bladder toxicity of Cytoxan. In the case of Rheumatrex (methotrexate), folic acid can be taken on a daily basis to minimize the side effects of this drug.

Certain measures to keep the complications in check, such as having your blood or platelet count checked regularly or liver enzyme studies done, are suggested. In addition, there may be dietary modifications that can help a patient to overcome the bad effects of these drugs. There are also wonderful new drugs that deal with side effects like nausea, vomiting, weakness, and cystitis. The advent of these drugs makes chemotherapy much easier to deal with. But remember that immunosuppressants are designed to be toxic, because that's how they'll do their intended job of suppression in the first place.

How do doctors monitor the patient
so that these complications are
least likely to occur?

Blood tests at specific intervals (such as every two weeks) that provide blood count information to monitor bone marrow function, frequent urinalyses, the monitoring of how long it takes for the blood to clot in certain cases, and regularly scheduled clinical exams are all useful in attempting to minimize complications. All of these procedures are mandatory in the case of chemotherapeutic treatments.

DHEA (DEHYDROEPIANDROSTERONE)

What is DHEA, and how is it related to lupus?

DHEA (dehydroepiandrosterone) is a male hormone metabolite. Male hormones are rapidly metabolized in women with lupus, although it is not known why. Because the change of male hormone metabolism is so pronounced in women with lupus, it was decided to investigate what would happen if the low levels of male hormones were replaced. Scientists decided to explore the possibility that replacing missing male hormones in female lupus patients might actually reverse the activity of the disease. As a result of that, more recent studies looked at the effects of certain male hormones on the clinical activity of the disease. Testosterone and other male hormones were tried. They had a major effect in reversing the illness but caused untoward side effects, including hairiness, big muscles, and deepening voice. The positive note is that one male hormone did not do that (unless it is used to excess)—DHEA. One way DHEA might work is it might be converted back into potent androgens in the body like testosterone.

Why is DHEA being investigated
so enthusiastically?

DHEA has the potential to have quite an impact on the medical world. First, unofficial data suggest that it does not produce unwanted side effects, such as excessive hair growth or big muscles. The only side effect that DHEA has been shown to have is acne, which occurs in about 5 percent of patients. Second, the drug seems to create a feeling of well-being, and some patients say it actually eliminates fatigue and the feeling of illness.

How does DHEA affect the immune system?

To date, there is not much known about the actual immune effects of this drug with regard to lupus. Most of the studies have been done in normal rats and mice and have investigated the metabolism of cytokines or interleukins. DHEA has distinct and beneficial effects on cytokines and interleukins that most investigators feel would be advantageous to patients who have lupus.

Is DHEA potentially beneficial to everyone who has lupus?

DHEA may be beneficial only to those patients with mild to moderate lupus. Patients with severe lupus do not seem to benefit as much. Although in some cases DHEA may cause them to feel a sense of well-being, their disease just flares on and can cause severe organ damage. It has not been shown that DHEA works to reverse the detrimental effects of severe disease or even to turn a flare around. The studies are not yet completed.

Is it possible that a future goal of aggressive treatment for flares or more severe manifestations of lupus will be to reduce the intensity of symptoms to the point where DHEA may then be effective?

Yes. It is possible that DHEA will be in the same activity class of drugs as the antimalarials like Plaquenil (hydroxychloroquine sulfate). In other words, it will only be used for mild to moderate disease. Not only may DHEA be given to patients with mild to moderate lupus, it may also be used in patients with more severe cases, who are being treated by drugs that are more potent. These patients may be given DHEA, in addition to the more potent drugs, to improve their sense of well-being.

Where can one get DHEA?

DHEA can be obtained in health food stores and certain pharmacies. But there is an important caution: it is still considered to be an experimental agent and is not approved for lupus at the time of this writing. Clinical trials of DHEA are still ongoing. One of the reasons that this caution is so important is because it is quite common among health-food advocates to use higher doses of many drugs that seem to be beneficial. But higher doses of an androgen can be detrimental and increase the possibility of severe side effects. Most studies find that dosages of DHEA should not exceed 200 milligrams per day. Another problem with DHEA is that because it's widely available, it's widely abused.

Are rheumatologists in a position to prescribe DHEA, or are only some working with it?

At the present time, DHEA is being used only experimentally at selected sites around the country for lupus treatment. These sites are sanctioned by the FDA (Food and Drug Administration) for its use. No rheumatologists are allowed to prescribe DHEA for lupus, rheumatoid arthritis, or any other disease. It is widely known, however, that many doctors in the field write prescriptions for DHEA on patient demand. But again, be aware that this is an experimental drug and that it is really inappropriate to use it at this time for this disease.

Q Given the potential benefits for large
numbers of people with lupus, what
would be involved in getting DHEA to
be approved so that it would no longer
be considered experimental?

Studies that are currently underway involve what are called phase 3 and
4 clinical trials that require that patients get the drug in a double-blind
process. A large group of patients meeting certain criteria is selected; one
half of the group is given the drug and the other half of the group is
given a placebo (sugar pill). The effects are then monitored by clinicians
and by laboratory testing, and it is determined which group achieved the
greatest improvement. If the group that has not taken the drug improves
as rapidly as those on the drug, then the drug is deemed to be ineffective. In a double-blind trial, the doctors treating the patients, the nurses
administering the drugs, and the patients in the experiment do not
know which group of patients is taking which agent. Once laboratory
results show scientific evidence of improvement as a result of DHEA,
the path toward FDA approval of the drug for lupus will be smoother.

OTHER MEDICATION ISSUES

Q Are there other medications, besides the
categories previously discussed, that can
be effective in lupus treatment?

Yes, but they are still experimental and not yet approved for use in lupus. Some of these drugs include male sex hormones; hormones that
turn off the pituitary; bromocriptine, which shuts off prolactin secretion; and monoclonal antibodies (laboratory-made antibodies) to eliminate specific cell populations like the CD4 helper population.

Why is it important to make sure to ask my doctor to give me the pneumococcal vaccine?

This vaccine protects the person from contracting disease from the pneumonia germ. In lupus, the spleen often becomes dysfunctional because it's clogged with immune complexes. This dysfunction, in essence, eliminates the spleen's ability to get rid of bacteria such as pneumococcus. Therefore, the vaccine is a must for lupus patients because it can protect them from getting *pneumococcal pneumonia*. There are other forms of infection for which the body relies on the spleen for clearance. Some of these infections are even more serious than the pneumococcus. Elimination of these bacteria is compromised because of the dysfunctional spleen.

Should someone with lupus be given flu shots?

The belief that flu shots given to patients with lupus would make the lupus worse once persisted; however, that is not the case. The influenza vaccine, provided it is weakened or killed, should be given to patients with lupus and can protect them against the flu just as it does anybody else. Since patients that are immunosuppressed with drugs can theoretically be sickened by live vaccine, it is better to give them a dead vaccine like the flu shot to keep them protected. There has never been a case of lupus induced by a vaccine, nor have lupus flares been activated by vaccines to our knowledge.

Why is it important for lupus patients to receive antibiotic protection for surgical procedures and other invasive procedures?

The reason we use antibiotic protection for lupus patients with heart problems and other medical concerns is that lupus patients often have vegetations on their heart valves, particularly if they have phospholipid antibodies and the antiphospholipid syndrome. Antibiotic protection (also called antibiotic prophylaxis) should be mandatory for such patients, especially when undergoing surgical procedures or invasive procedures like dental work, because the antibiotics protect them from infection. There is also a danger of these lupus patients being infected with organisms because many of them are being immunosuppressed with steroids or chemotherapy.

Why is it important for lupus patients to get prompt treatment of any infections with antibiotics?

The prompt treatment of any infections with antibiotics is important because most patients with lupus are immunosuppressed; therefore, their defenses are down. The prompt treatment of infections with antibiotics prevents them from getting very sick or even dying of the infection. Remember, twenty years ago, the most common cause of death in lupus was infection. Certain antibiotics, however, like sulfa drugs, often cause terrible allergic reactions in lupus patients and are to be avoided.

Why is it so often recommended that if one
is on prednisone one's dosage should
be increased if one is undergoing a
surgical procedure?

That's because the adrenal glands, when they are functioning normally, secrete increased amounts of cortisone during stressful periods. When a patient is on prednisone, the adrenal glands are suppressed and are not able to produce their own natural dose of cortisone. Over long periods of time, the adrenal glands even shrink. So it is necessary to raise the amount of steroids that lupus patients are taking to compensate for the reduced production of the adrenal glands. This protects the body from the stress of whatever procedure is being performed.

Why are certain categories of drugs
sometimes used in combination
with others?

When drugs are given to treat lupus patients, the idea is to achieve maximum immune suppression for that patient without causing undue harm. It is sometimes necessary to use drugs together, like prednisone and Imuran (azathioprine), prednisone and Plaquenil (hydroxychloroquine sulfate), or prednisone and Cytoxan (cyclophosphamide). Many different combinations of drugs can be used to treat this disease.

Are drugs effective in controlling lupus?

There are always drugs that can be used to control lupus. There are also maneuvers that can be used to treat the disease, such as bed rest and the prevention of flares. However, one must always remember that they must be used under a doctor's care, and the doctor's instructions must be followed to the letter in order for treatment to be both safe and effec-

tive. Many patients feel that they can monitor their own drug therapy.
This is not the case.

What is an antipyretic?

A drug or agent that will lower a fever. Drugs of this variety are aspirin,
NSAIDs, and Tylenol (acetaminophen).

When are diuretics used in the treatment of lupus?

Diuretics (medications to eliminate water from the body) are generally used
when a person is full of fluid and experiences edema, or water around
the lungs or ankles. There are many causes. Most of these are related to
the heart. However, it is very common for lupus patients to have edema
as a result of low serum proteins that were lost through the kidneys.

When are antihypertensive drugs used?

Antihypertensive drugs are used when blood pressure is high. Elevated
blood pressure is common in patients with lupus for a variety of reasons,
including damaged kidneys, problems with the heart, vasospasm (spasms
in the blood vessels, reducing blood flow), or use of drugs that are
known to raise blood pressure.

What role can one's pharmacist play in helping one with his or her medication?

Your pharmacist can tell you which medications are dangerous, which
should be monitored carefully by your physician, and which interact
with other agents that you may be taking.

Is it okay to use generic medication?

Absolutely—although all medications should be used only under a doctor's care.

Is there a time limit for how long a person suffering from lupus should take medication?

No. The amount and strength of medication depends largely on the extent of one's disease.

Can a person taking medication consume alcohol?

Alcohol in moderate amounts is generally all right, although it depends on the medication you are taking. However, you must remember that alcohol reacts with just about everything. The power of anti-inflammatory drugs can be increased by alcohol, or it might interfere with, or increase the toxic effects of, some of the chemotherapeutic drugs being given to lupus patients. Always check with your doctor before consuming alcohol while on any medication.

6.

THE IMPACT OF LUPUS

· ·

Lupus can have an impact on virtually every aspect of your life. In order to live with it most effectively, you should know the ways it can affect you as well as what you can do to better deal with it. This chapter includes questions about the variety of ways lupus can affect your life, as well as answers indicating how you can improve your quality of life.

ACTIVITIES AND DAILY CONCERNS

How can lupus affect activities of daily living?

Daily activities are affected by lupus pain, insomnia, extreme fatigue, depression, the unpredictability of lupus, medication, and poor body image. These problems can lead to lower self-esteem and mood swings. Many people with lupus have much greater difficulty taking care of themselves or their children.

What can I do around the house to conserve my energy?

Some ways of conserving energy are to rest or take naps if possible, to ask for help, to prioritize what you have to do (as well as what you *want* to do), to place things within easy reach, and so on.

Are there some people who cannot work because of lupus?

Yes, due to both physical and psychological symptoms. Physical symptoms can include extreme fatigue or pain. Psychological symptoms may include concentration problems (due to an affected central nervous system) or depression.

Does one have any recourse if fired because of lupus?

Yes. The Americans With Disabilities Act states that you cannot be fired if you are adequately doing your job. No employer has the right to fire you simply because you have lupus. So if you have any doubts about your situation, consult an attorney who specializes in this area.

Should I tell my employer that I have lupus?

Each case is different. Sometimes you should, and sometimes it may not be a good idea. This depends on the company and administration. You are not required to tell everything about your illness, but lying on your application for employment can be grounds for discharge.

How can I educate my employer and colleagues about lupus?

If people are receptive, you can give them helpful books, pamphlets, or other reading materials about lupus. Check the appendix for a list of suggested books. If they are not receptive, take your time, be patient, and show them how well you're handling lupus.

How does lupus affect school performance?

School performance may be affected by extreme fatigue, pain, or central nervous system involvement, which can cause memory and concentration difficulties or even seizures.

Are there any sports or other recreational activities in which lupus patients cannot participate?

Remember that all people with lupus are different. Sports or other recreational activities that some lupus patients may need to avoid include ones that are predominantly outdoors (in order to minimize sun exposure), require a great deal of energy to be exerted, or present a situation in which there is a good chance of breaking bones.

Is there any reason why I can't travel because of lupus?

Unless you are experiencing a flare and need to be near your doctor, there is no particular reason why one needs to avoid traveling. There are doctors in every country of the world who are familiar with SLE.

Q Should I make any special arrangements
    if I travel?

Arrange to secure the names of rheumatologists (and hospitals, if it makes you feel more secure) in the area of your destination, in advance.

Q Does insurance cover the treatment of lupus?

Most insurance plans cover some of the cost but usually not all of it.

Q Do Medicaid and Medicare cover the
    treatment of lupus?

Both Medicaid and Medicare provide some coverage of lupus treatment. But many doctors do not accept Medicaid, and Medicare often pays so little of it that the patient's copayment is often quite high.

Q What happens when one switches jobs but
    can't get insurance at the new job?

This is a major problem with today's insurance industry. If you switch jobs and cannot get insurance at your new job, by law you are entitled to continue to pay for your old insurance for up to eighteen months. The problem is, of course, that this can be very expensive, and you still have to worry about obtaining new insurance.

Can lupus patients obtain Social Security benefits?

Although one would think that living with lupus is a clear basis for obtaining Social Security benefits, this has been a very difficult area for many lupus patients. Often people are denied the first time they apply for benefits, and many are even denied when they appeal. In some cases, people retain disability lawyers. Documentation is required from all your doctors, and most of the time it is necessary to see an "impartial" physician. The good news is that once disability is approved, the benefits are paid retroactively to the date of your first application.

SEX

How can lupus interfere with sexual activity?

People with lupus can experience considerable lack of energy, a loss of sex drive, and pain during sexual activity. Some female patients with lupus can experience irritation and dryness around the vagina due to a lack of vaginal glandular secretion. This problem, often occurring in Sjogren's syndrome or sicca syndrome—syndromes that may occur with lupus—can cause intercourse to be quite painful. Pain in the joints can also cause problems. Lupus rashes can also occur in the most inconvenient places and result in considerable irritation. Mouth or vaginal ulcers or sores can interfere with sexual activities, in terms of both physical discomfort and desire.

Certain medications may also contribute to sexual problems, including pain killers, sedatives and tranquilizers, and alcohol. Small amounts of these medications can increase feelings of relaxation too much, thereby inhibiting a fully aroused sexual state. Certain antihypertensive medications can have a direct negative effect on sexual desire.

What can be done to improve one's sex life?

There are many things that can improve one's sex life. Adequate treatment can result in an increase in energy and sex drive. Procedures that can help relax any muscles used during sex or that reduce pain can be helpful (such as moist heat, warm baths, or compresses). Limbering up, or stretching, exercises can also facilitate more comfortable sexual experiences. Aerobic exercise can even help. Different positions may better facilitate sex. Using pillows or knee pads can decrease discomfort by putting less of a strain on uncomfortable joints.

Aspirin and other medication can help joint pain, Raynaud's phenomenon, Sjogren's syndrome, and other symptoms that can decrease sexual pleasure. There are lubricant creams on the market that can be applied to the vagina to make sexual intercourse more comfortable. Joint and muscle pains can be treated with either an anti-inflammatory or a steroid. Treatment for mouth or vaginal ulcers can help improve sexual functioning. Treatments include steroid applications, such as special mouthwashes with added antibiotics, for mouth ulcers and steroid suppositories for vaginal ulcers.

What role do psychological factors play in one's sex life?

One cannot ignore the role that psychological factors play in sexual difficulties. A decreased interest in sex, concerns about self-esteem, a negative body image, concerns about strains put on the relationship, and self-consciousness can all interfere with sexual satisfaction. Working these problems out with your partner can often do a lot to improve sexual functioning. Consulting a professional for help may be beneficial if other strategies for improvement do not work.

What types of birth control are most appropriate for people with lupus?

The answer to this question is still quite controversial. Most experts believe that, at the present time, birth control should be limited to condoms and spermicidal jelly or creams, or a diaphragm.

Are there any types of birth control that should be avoided?

Contraceptives containing estrogen have not yet been proven safe and should be avoided. One preliminary research study has suggested that women who take birth control pills early in life are twice as likely to later get lupus than those who started them later in life or do not take them at all. At the present time, it is not believed to be safe for lupus patients to take birth control pills. More data is needed, and research into their hormonal effects is in progress.

Can female lupus patients take hormones after menopause?

The use of hormone replacement therapy (HRT) is a controversial issue for women with lupus, but it is less of an issue than taking birth control pills before menopause. There are a number of controlled federal studies in progress to answer the question about the use of pills in menopause. At the present time, most experts believe that women who have had total hysterectomies and those in menopause can use estrogen replacement therapy, provided that the average levels of estrogen for premenopausal women are not exceeded.

PREGNANCY

Is there any concern about lupus patients getting pregnant?

There are most certainly problems with being pregnant with lupus. Most women with lupus can have a healthy baby if they follow two simple rules. Make sure that your disease is under control prior to becoming pregnant (if the pregnancy is planned), and have your doctor carefully monitor your pregnancy with frequent exams. Sometimes it is difficult to predict when you are going to get pregnant. Many patients with lupus have trouble becoming pregnant because of either the disease activity or medication. There is no danger in being on certain drugs when you get pregnant, but others may be dangerous. The important thing is to consult your doctor immediately so that he or she can give you advice about what to do with various medications.

How might lupus affect one's pregnancy?

Lupus is usually more detrimental if it is active prior to conception. Patients can have a stillbirth, or they can develop *toxemia of pregnancy.* Toxemia of pregnancy, also called *preeclampsia,* can cause such things as high blood pressure, swelling, and transient diabetes—diabetes that comes and goes during pregnancy. The reason that lupus patients have a propensity to develop it is unknown. Toxemia of pregnancy can be dangerous because it can cause spontaneous abortions, or it can cause the patient to have strokes, among other problems.

Patients with renal disease and with antiphospholipid antibodies have to be especially vigilant. For reasons that are not clear, patients with kidney disease can become very sick during pregnancy. This probably has to do with abnormal fluid shifts from the blood vessels to the tissues surrounding the blood vessels, causing edema; blood pressure changes; and increased weight caused by their kidney problems. Kidney function can go downhill without expert medical care during this time. Patients who have antiphospholipid antibodies run the risk of their blood clotting during pregnancy. It is believed that the blood is more coagulable during pregnancy.

Can one's pregnancy affect the course of lupus?

Yes. In some cases, pregnancy can worsen symptoms or even trigger a lupus flare. In other cases, pregnancy can bring about a remission. The reasons for these changes are not yet fully understood, but they are probably due to the sudden changes in the hormones during the course of pregnancy.

How can a woman with lupus ensure a safe pregnancy?

It is important to have careful examinations by an obstetrician/gynecologist familiar with lupus, and to see your rheumatologist frequently. Make sure your doctors routinely conduct urinalyses, blood pressure checks, coagulation tests, and blood sugar analyses.

Is it wrong to become pregnant if your lupus is active?

It is prudent to try not to become pregnant at this time. Depressions in the complement values or a rise in the abnormal renal chemicals like creatinine and blood urea nitrogen may lead to problems for the mother and the fetus.

Are there any statistics as to how often lupus pregnancy is problem free?

No. There are no reliable statistics at this point. This may be because there are so many variables involved, including the degree of lupus activity in the mother and the treatment used.

What are the causes of pregnancy complications with lupus?

No one really knows. The most recent discussions center around micro emboli, or small clots, from lupus anticoagulants in the placenta (from which the baby derives its nourishment). Other theories predict that the antibodies have a direct toxic effect on the placenta and the fetus. Some theories also focus on the fact that the vacillation of hormones in the mother directly affects the state of the mother's immune system—estrogens raise the levels of antibodies, and testosterone lowers the levels.

Are lupus sufferers more prone to prolonged morning sickness?

The incidence of morning sickness in lupus mothers has never been studied. If a lupus patient suffers from prolonged morning sickness, it may be caused by high levels of estrogen; on the other hand, it might be the result of high levels of cytokines or interleukins, as these might affect any pregnant woman.

Will a lupus patient without a skin rash develop one after becoming pregnant?

It's possible. Pregnancy can bring out many new lupus symptoms. Other symptoms that can be affected by pregnancy include arthritis, muscle weakness, and inflammation of the heart muscles or linings of the lungs.

What is high-risk pregnancy?

A high-risk pregnancy is when there is possible danger to either the mother or the baby. Usually a high-risk pregnancy requires weekly or biweekly physical checkups to ensure that things are going well with mother and fetus. Pregnant patients with lupus are always considered to be high risk.

What complications should doctors most carefully watch for during pregnancy?

High blood pressure, high blood sugar, abnormal urine sediments, slow heartbeat in the baby, and overall worsening of the disease in the mother are all things that doctors should watch out for during routine exams—as they should during any pregnancy.

What are the chances of the baby developing lupus?

The chances of the baby actually developing lupus are very, very small. In neonatal lupus, the mother's antibodies temporarily pass through the placenta to the baby. These antibodies can cause the baby to develop a severe rash, or, in rare cases, a heart block (the heart does not beat because the conduction system of the heart is blocked) that will require the baby to wear a pacemaker to get the heart to beat normally. The rash is usually transient, but the heart block can be permanent.

Which medications are acceptable during pregnancy?

The most important, powerful immunosuppressant medication that can be taken during pregnancy is prednisone. There is no evidence that prednisone has any adverse effects during pregnancy. Heparin, a blood thinner, is another important drug that can be taken during pregnancy. Drugs like Cytoxan (cyclophosphamide); Leukeran (chlorambucil); and Coumadin (crystalline warfarin sodium), a blood thinner, must *never* be taken during pregnancy. These drugs should even be discontinued before conception, when possible. However, most patients cannot predict when they are going to become pregnant, so it is best to consult with your physician for advice on what to start and stop and when.

So prednisone has no effect on a developing fetus?

None. Passage of prednisone across the placenta is minimal. Patients taking large dosages of cortisone can even safely breastfeed, as the amount of prednisone in breast milk is minimal.

Is Plaquenil safe to take during pregnancy?

Although there have been relatively few human pregnancy studies involving the use of Plaquenil (hydroxychloroquine sulfate), several recent reports state that the use of this drug is quite safe and that many healthy babies have been born from mothers taking this agent. However, it would be wise to consult with an expert, if this is an issue of concern for you.

What is the relationship between anticardiolipin antibodies and miscarriages?

It is suggested that lupus patients who have had more than one miscarriage have more antiphospholipid antibodies (such as anticardiolipin antibodies) than patients who do not have antiphospholipid antibodies. The reasons for this are not known. Various theories include clotting of the vessels to the placenta or a direct action of the antibody on the placenta itself.

How does lupus affect menstruation?

Patients with lupus can become *amenorrheic* (ceased menstruation) or *oligomenorrheic* (having scanty periods) or they can bleed very heavily. Lupus patients' disease can worsen during certain times in their menstrual cycle. This is probably due to fluctuating sex hormones.

PSYCHOLOGICAL FACTORS

Why do people become depressed because of lupus?

People become depressed for many reasons—the pain, fatigue, side effects from medication (which, in addition to directly causing depression, can also lead to depression because they can cause weight gain, loss of hair where you want it, and growth of hair where you don't want it), and required lifestyle changes. In addition, many people with lupus look well, so others have a hard time believing they are really sick. Some people lose friends because they often have to cancel appointments at the last minute. People with lupus may become depressed because of difficulties carrying out their accustomed roles (parental, marital, social, and so on). In some cases, depression in the patient with lupus might actually be due to biochemical causes, directly due to medication or other biochemical changes or deficiencies, or hormonal changes.

What mental changes can take place because of depression?

When you are depressed, you are much more likely to think negative thoughts, including feelings of uselessness and worthlessness, not caring about others or yourself, and feeling as if your family would be better off without you. Suicidal thoughts may occur because of worries that you'll never get better. Other mental changes include the inability to sleep (actually quite common in lupus), low self-esteem, and engaging in obsessive activity, such as overeating.

What are the physical consequences of depression?

Depression can actually cause a flare of the disease.

What can be done to treat depression?

Depression often responds to psychotherapy, and this is the best recommendation. It is most important that the therapist have some familiarity with lupus. In severe cases, it may be necessary to obtain prescriptions for antidepressant drugs.

Can deep bouts of depression or even mental illness be a result of lupus?

Absolutely. Some 67 percent of patients with lupus have psychological abnormalities. These range from neurotic problems to actual psychosis, and can often be related to central nervous system involvement.

Q Why do so many lupus patients blame
      everything that goes wrong with them
      on lupus?

This is due to a lack of knowledge of exactly what lupus can and cannot affect. Both patients and physicians may be guilty of this.

Q What is it about lupus that causes anger?

People with lupus are often angry. Lupus patients may be angry because
their previous life has been taken away, their future life is not what they
had planned, family and friends do not understand the illness, they lose
friends, they cannot work or take care of their family, they feel that their
only contact with the outside world is in the doctor's office (where they
wait for long periods of time, are often mistreated by the staff, and may
not be satisfied with the doctor). Often people with lupus experience
the "Why me?" syndrome, which can create feelings of anger.

Q What causes anxiety?

Lupus can cause much anxiety—uncertainty about your medical future,
as well as the future of your family, social relationships, and job. You
worry about whether the treatments and/or medicine will work. You
may be anxious about developing additional symptoms or problems, or
even about dying from lupus. Often, however, the main source of anxiety is lack of knowledge about the disease, as mentioned earlier, so it
makes sense to learn as much as you can.

Q Why is it important to avoid getting
      overly anxious?

Anxiety can create enough stress to cause a flare.

What causes guilt?

The thought of the emotional "pain" that your disease might cause others can create a fair amount of guilt. For example, you may fear that your spouse is stuck with a partner who is sick and cannot lead a "normal" life, that the illness is expensive and you may have to leave your job, that you cannot take care of your family the way other parents can, that your spouse will have to do more than other spouses do, and that you may be passing the gene for the illness on to your children. In addition, the lower quality of life and the many complaints that lupus patients have cause them guilt.

What can be done about these negative emotions?

Anger, anxiety, and guilt are just a few of the negative emotions that may be experienced by lupus patients. It is important (for both physical and psychological reasons) to work to improve your emotional state. As with depression, psychotherapy can help. Learning relaxation techniques (such as deep breathing, meditation, and visualization) and changing negative thinking to more realistic, positive thinking can help. Working with a professional who is trained in effective coping techniques of this nature has helped many people who otherwise would have a much harder time dealing with their disease.

Why do mood swings sometimes occur in people with lupus?

Mood swings are not unusual. They can be due to the central nervous system being affected. Mood swings can also result from the feelings of illness that vacillate from day to day. For example, if you feel well, your mood may be better than it would be if you were experiencing a great deal of pain.

What kind of impact does lupus have on other family members?

This often depends on the knowledge that other family members have about the disease. Many families are devastated by the disease, their fear of it, and the potential effects they believe might result from childbirth or marriage. They may be affected by the fact that roles in the family may have to totally change—for example, the spouse and children may have to take over for the sick parent, or parents may have to care for adult children. A united family can be a valuable asset for a lupus patient. If lupus causes problems within the family, efforts should be made (either with or without professional help) to eliminate these problems for the sake of the health of the lupus patient.

How helpful are support groups in the treatment of lupus?

Support groups can play a very important role in living with lupus. People may find groups helpful so that they don't feel as isolated as before. Participants can share their feelings of frustration, anger, or guilt. A good support group can be very helpful in providing facts and suggestions to help people to better cope with lupus.

THE ROLE OF THE PHYSICIAN

Why is a good doctor-patient relationship so important in lupus?

The physician must have an intimate knowledge of his or her patient's illness in order to provide the proper treatment on a timely basis, as well as to alleviate any concerns.

What can I do to make the most of this relationship?

Understand that doctors are only human. Lupus is a disease demanding much attention, and a delicate balance exists between patient and doctor. It can be very helpful to keep records of everything you take and of every symptom you experience, and to keep all of your medical records in one place. In the event of an emergency or when you are away from home, it may be important for your records to be faxed or sent to the hospital or doctor who is trying to treat you. Work with your physician.

When is it most appropriate to contact my physician?

Whenever a new sign or symptom is causing discomfort, or when you feel that it may be necessary to modify your drug dosages, it's time to call the doctor.

What are some of the symptoms that should be reported immediately to the doctor?

Many signs and symptoms are important. However, clinical experience tells us that the following are among the most significant: sudden shortness of breath, numbness or tingling in a hand or foot, blood in the stool or urine, chest pain, and fever.

What are some of the things I should be able to take care of on my own?

Symptoms with which you are familiar rarely require an emergency visit. However, no new symptom should be overlooked with lupus.

How should I deal with a physician who
 is not handling things the way
 I would like him or her to?

Discuss this with your doctor. If nothing changes, get a second opinion, and if necessary, change physicians.

Why is it sometimes necessary
 to get a second opinion?

Getting a second opinion from another doctor can often give patients new insight or new therapeutic options to consider.

CONCLUSION

. . . .

A tremendous amount has been learned about lupus in the recent past. Although you may not always hear about them, a multitude of studies about lupus are being carried out all over the world. The major issue being investigated today is the cause of immune dysfunction. The reasons for more females than males having lupus, the "hereditary nature" of the disease, and other aspects, such as the origin and function of phospholipid antibodies, are also all current areas of research interest. The hope is that this research will continue to shed more and more light on the disease, its cause(s), its treatments, and ultimately, its cure. Although there are many exciting, promising discoveries on the horizon, it is hoped that by the time the next edition of this book is published, more of those valuable findings will be included as fact.

Our intent throughout the book is to focus on what is known and what has been learned about lupus. Individuals living with lupus are becoming their own best advocates as they become more knowledgeable about the disease. It is hoped that this book will provide a lot of the information that will help in that regard.

While it may be difficult to answer everyone's questions about every aspect of lupus, we are sensitive to the importance of getting up-to-date information and will continue to research the latest answers to significant issues for those living with lupus. We invite you, our readers, to contact us, in care of the publisher, with any questions you would like us to consider for inclusion in the next edition of this book. Meanwhile, living with lupus is a day-in, day-out struggle. We wish you the best in your efforts to succeed in this endeavor.

Appendix

For further information, contact:

Lupus Foundation of America
200 L Street, NW
Washington, D.C. 20036
1-800-558-0121
1-202-349-1155

FOR FURTHER READING

Aladjem, H. *Understanding Lupus.* New York: Scribner's, 1985.

Aladjem, H., and Schur, P. *In Search of the Sun.* New York: Scribner's, 1988.

Butler, B. *The Monster Under the Bed.* St. Louis: Lupus Foundation of America, Missouri Chapter, 1989.

Carr, R. *Lupus Erythematosus: A Handbook for Physicians, Patients, and Their Families.* Washington, D.C.: Lupus Foundation of America, 1986.

Lahita, R. G. *Systemic Lupus Erythematosus.* 2nd ed. New York: Churchill Livingstone, 1992.

———. *Systemic Lupus Erythematosus.* 3rd ed. San Diego: Academic Press, 1998.

Lewis, K. *Successful Living with Chronic Illness.* New York: Avery, 1985.

Phillips, R. *Control Your Pain! 144 Sure-Fire Strategies for Reducing the Pain of Lupus.* New York: Balance, 1996.

———. *Coping with Lupus.* New York: Avery, 1991.

———. *Living Well . . . Despite Lupus! 204 Sure-Fire Techniques for Taking Charge of Your Life.* New York: Balance, 1996.

———. *Successful Living with Lupus: A Balance Strategy Guidebook.* New York: Balance, 2000.

Pitzele, S. *We Are Not Alone.* New York: Workman, 1986.

Wallace, D. *The Lupus Book.* New York: Oxford University Press, 1995.

Index

About the Authors

Robert Lahita, M.D., Ph.D., FACP, FACR, FRCP, is Professor of Medicine at New York Medical College and the Chairman of Medicine at the new Liberty-Health Center in New Jersey, which is part of the Mount Sinai Medical School. Formerly Chief of Rheumatology and Connective Tissue Diseases at Saint Vincent's Hospital in New York City, he serves as Senior Attending Physician at Saint Vincent's Medical Center and the Jersey City Medical Center, in New Jersey.

Dr. Lahita is a fellow of the American College of Physicians, the American College of Rheumatology, and the Royal College of Physicians. He is also President of the Seventh International Congress on Lupus and Related Diseases, held in New York City in 2004.

Internationally recognized for his clinical research in systemic lupus erythematosus, Dr. Lahita's findings have been the subject of more than 140 published articles and book chapters, and he is the editor of the standard textbook called *Systemic Lupus Erythematosus* (fourth edition in press). Dr. Lahita also serves as the editor of the *Yearbook of Rheumatology* and the Associate Editor of the journal *Lupus,* and he is a reviewer for numerous medical journals, including *The Lancet, Arthritis and Rheumatism,* and *New England Journal of Medicine,* among others. In addition to his work with academic publications, Dr. Lahita has written three books for the general public, *Rheumatoid Arthritis: Everything You Need to Know, The Arthritis Solution,* and *Women and Autoimmunity.*

Robert H. Phillips, Ph.D., is a practicing psychologist in Long Island, New York. He is the founder and director of the Center for Coping, a multiservice organization that helps individuals with medical, emotional, and family problems. He is actively involved with a number of local and national medical organizations, including the Lupus Foundation of America, the Arthritis Foundation, and the American Autoimmune Related Diseases Association.

Dr. Phillips is the author of more than thirty books as well as numerous articles on a variety of subjects in psychology, and has appeared on local and national radio and television programs. He continues to lecture at conventions, universities, and professional meetings throughout the country.